KU-164-168

Culture, communication and nursing

Philip Burnard, PhD, RN
Cardiff University

Paul Gill, PhD, RN
University of Glamorgan

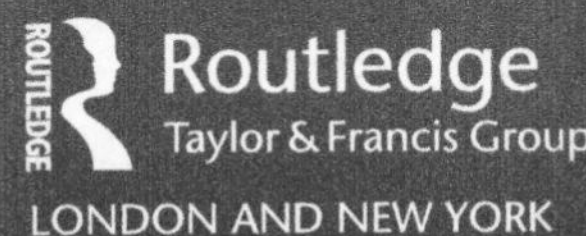

Routledge
Taylor & Francis Group
LONDON AND NEW YORK

First published 2008 by Pearson Education Limited

Published 2013 by Routledge
2 Park Square, Milton Park, Abingdon, Oxon OX14 4RN
711 Third Avenue, New York, NY 10017, USA

Routledge is an imprint of the Taylor & Francis Group, an informa business

Copyright © 2009, Taylor & Francis.

The rights of Philip Burnard and Paul Gill to be identified as authors of this work have been asserted by them in accordance with the Copyright, Designs and Patents Act 1988.

All rights reserved. No part of this book may be reprinted or reproduced or utilised in any form or by any electronic, mechanical, or other means, now known or hereafter invented, including photocopying and recording, or in any information storage or retrieval system, without permission in writing from the publishers.

Notices
Knowledge and best practice in this field are constantly changing. As new research and experience broaden our understanding, changes in research methods, professional practices, or medical treatment may become necessary.

Practitioners and researchers must always rely on their own experience and knowledge in evaluating and using any information, methods, compounds, or experiments described herein. In using such information or methods they should be mindful of their own safety and the safety of others, including parties for whom they have a professional responsibility.

To the fullest extent of the law, neither the Publisher nor the authors, contributors, or editors, assume any liability for any injury and/or damage to persons or property as a matter of products liability, negligence or otherwise, or from any use or operation of any methods, products, instructions, or ideas contained in the material herein.

ISBN 13: 978-0-13-232892-0 (pbk)

British Library Cataloguing-in-Publication Data
A catalogue record for this book is available from the British Library

Library of Congress Cataloging-in-Publication Data
Burnard, Philip.
Culture, communication and nursing / Philip Burnard, Paul Gill.
p. ; cm.
Includes bibliographical references.
ISBN 978-0-13-232892-0 (pbk.)
1. Transcultural nursing. 2. Communication in nursing. I. Gill, Paul (Paul Wyndham), 1971- II. Title.
[DNLM: 1. Transcultural Nursing. 2. Communication. 3. Nursing Theory. WY 107 B963c 2008]
RT86.54.B87 2008
610.73--dc22

2008035583

Typeset in 9/13 Interstate by Macmillan Publishing Solutions

Contents

Acknowledgements

Philip Burnard

Many people have contributed both directly and indirectly to this book. First, as always, I thank my family, Sally, Aaron and Becky, for their support. I would also like to thank Dr Sandy Kirkman, Una Hebden and Linda Thomas for all their help.

In Thailand, there are too many people to name individually, but particular thanks go to Dr Wassana Naiyapatana and Dr Ong-Art Naiyapatana. Both have given freely of their time, and the former and I have been research colleagues for more 10 years. I consider myself lucky to have such helpful and valuable friends. Thanks and good wishes also go to Narakorn Kreokhamla, from whom I learned a huge amount about Thai culture and the Thai world view. I would also like to thank all the people, both students and teachers, I have met at a considerable number of Thai universities and who have shared with me something of their culture. Similarly, I thank my colleagues in Brunei for their time and patience in letting me know more about both Islam and about Bruneian nursing. I have been associated with the School of Nursing in Brunei for 17 years and have learned a great deal. My particular thanks, there, go to Hasnan Kahan.

Finally, I would like to thank all at Pearson Education, who have always been supportive. In particular, I wish to thank Kate Brewin, who supported me through my uncertain start to this book and showed considerable patience in the preparation of it.

Paul Gill

First and foremost I would like to thank Phil for providing me with the opportunity to co-write the book, and for his encouragement and support throughout the process. Like Phil, I would also like to thank Kate Brewin and all at Pearson Education for their support. I am very grateful to my colleagues at the University of Glamorgan, who were kind enough to write some of the case studies in the book, based on their personal experiences. Last, but not least, I would like to thank my wife Lisa, for her patience, encouragement and support.

Publisher's Acknowledgements

We would like to thank the following reviewers for their helpful and constructive comments that have helped shaped the book:

Frank Milligan, University of Bedfordshire

Helen C. Walsh, Swansea University

Julia Pridmore, Swansea University

Introduction

There are many roads to truth and no culture has a corner in the path or is better equipped than others to search for it. ***Edward Hall***

We express aspects of our culture every day. Whenever we communicate with others, we demonstrate our beliefs, values, thoughts, feelings and attitudes – all things that have arisen out of the culture (or cultures) in which we have been born or raised. Nursing is now a cross-cultural affair in many countries, particularly in the United Kingdom, and this book is aimed mostly at a readership in that country. However, as always in reading books written from different perspectives, it should also be of value to those who live outside the UK. We can gain much by reading 'particular' points of view. In reading about other cultures, and even more by living in them, we can understand more about our own. By nursing patients, and working with health professionals from other cultures and communicating with them, we can also learn a great deal about their beliefs and behaviours, provided we are both observant and open minded.

With regard to the latter, we immediately come across a particular problem in the culture debate: most of us, if we do not think carefully about it, feel that *our* way of thinking and *our* culture are somehow more 'right' than those of other countries. This is known in the literature as ethnocentricity, and will be discussed later. The danger, perhaps, comes when we confuse what we *believe* with what is *true*. Any amount of believing something does not make it a fact.

In passing, we should note that even a country as small as the UK has a variety of cultures. Those who live in Scotland, Wales or Northern Ireland would not necessarily demonstrate the same cultural practices as are found in England. Furthermore, there are often regional cultural differences within each country, and also often religious and language differences too. With governmental control from a central UK parliament being increasingly devolved to Wales, Scotland and Northern Ireland, it seems likely that degrees of separate culture will increase. This creation of smaller countries is happening in other parts of the world too. Consider, for example, the way in which the country that was called the USSR (Union of Soviet Socialist Republics) has been split into a very considerable number of smaller, reasonably independent republics.

East and West

There is often a tendency, when discussing cultures, to divide the world into East and West, as if those two areas were individually homogenous, but there are a number of problems with this. The first is geographical: given that the world is round, 'east and west' have meaning only according to the point where you are standing. If you are in Japan, then the US is east and Hong Kong is west. And how would we place Australia? Second, many people in those countries we think of as east consider the US and the UK (being in the west) to be very similar. Anyone living in and/or visiting those countries will know that this is not the case. Similarly, India and China are considered to be in the east, but their cultures are very different from each other. Historically, the division into east and west probably arose during the times when the UK and other northern European countries colonised many other countries, and therefore East and West refer to points east and west of the UK and Europe.

This division also has implications for nursing. It is easy to fall into the trap of considering some of the patients we care for as 'eastern', despite the fact that they may come from a huge and wide-ranging array of cultures. Similarly, in nurse education, 'overseas' students are sometimes grouped together as if they had more in common than having come from different countries.

Some recent writers on the issue have suggested that a more accurate division is between Islam and the West, or tradition and obedience versus modernity and liberalism (Harris, 2006). Again, the division is not a particularly helpful one, for a number of reasons. First, the West, in this categorisation, is not made up of countries and cultures that are all the same (the US, for example, is far more obviously 'Christian' than the UK and parts of northern Europe). Second, not all of the countries that are not in the west are Islamic: Thailand is Buddhist, and China is mostly atheistic. Similarly, Russia, a huge country, is made up of a mixture of republics, some of which are Islamic and some of which are not. Given the world events that are taking place at the time of writing, it is important for all of us to understand as completely as we can the cultural differences that make up the world.

However, we have to have some way of being able to talk about differences of culture, and in this book we are sometimes going to refer to east and west, if only as shorthand. It is important, though, to note that we are not automatically generalising and suggesting that 'everyone in the east is like this', or that 'all those people who live in the west believe this'. As always, we must be on our guard against over-generalising cultural values. It is quite possible to imagine giving a talk to a group of people from the UK or from China and a number of the audience saying 'Well, I am not like that'. Alongside our cultural inheritance also goes the fact of our consciousness: the fact that we can *choose* to be different. Culture, then, is not a set of rules but more a set of influences that help to shape people and society.

We also use the division of east and west for another reason. For the past 10 years, the first author has being doing cultural research about communication, stress and mental health care in Thailand. In many ways, Thai culture is about as different from UK culture as it is possible to imagine. We will therefore use various relevant examples from some of this Thai research to illustrate and to compare and contrast different aspects of communication in nursing, in the two countries. We will also offer a report of some of that research to further highlight those differences.

For many in the UK, Thailand is a sunny and beautiful tourist destination. It is, of course, also very many other things. It is a country that has never been colonised – unlike many of its neighbours; it is considered to be a third-world country but enjoys a high standard of education and health care; there is considerable corruption; it is ruled by the longest-reigning monarch in the world. Its capital, Bangkok, is a thriving metropolis, not dissimilar to Hong Kong or New York, but with its own distinct 'Thainess'. Thai culture is very polite and hierarchical, with an emphasis on respect for other people. Thailand is also a country of extremes, with huge numbers of people living in or near poverty, and a few very rich people. These and many other reasons make it a country very different from those that make up the UK. It is, then, an ideal country for highlighting differences in culture. We use it in this book to illustrate nursing and communication differences in two different cultural settings. The intention is not to highlight Thailand as a place to live or work, but to help you - as we suggest above - to think about cultural issues as they relate to nursing and communication. To offer a third and yet again different culture, we also draw on research from Brunei, a small Muslim sultanate. Understanding culture can probably only come from comparisons. Here, we compare three very different cultural settings.

Communication in Nursing

A great deal of our work as nurses involves communication. We communicate daily with patients, other nurses, other health-care staff, relatives and the general public. How we do so will depend to some degree on our level in a hierarchy, for example a first-year student nurse or a senior sister. How we react to junior and senior staff, to relatives and to patients often depends on our status. Whereas in the UK this hierarchy is not particularly marked (although it would be wrong to assume that it did not exist), it is very important in some other cultures and countries. In many South-east Asian cultures, for example, first-year students are very junior in comparison to second-year ones, and have to show respect for their senior student colleagues.

Similarly, patients occupy part of the hierarchy and communication with them will depend on their perceived place in it. In British culture there is sometimes a tendency to 'infantilise' older people and to treat them rather like children. Again, as we shall see, this would not be the case in some other cultures, where older people are held in very high respect. Patients themselves, if they come from different cultures, will hold nurses, doctors and other health-care workers in varying degrees of regard. In some cultures, only the doctor's word is important: nurses are seen as very much on the lower rung of the hierarchy. In other cultures, nurses are respected as professionals in their own right. What we cannot do, as nurses, is to assume that all of our patients will view us in the same light.

We might also note differences in status and hence differences in communication styles between private and public hospitals. In private hospitals, where the patient is paying directly for his or her care, they may (or may not) be treated more deferentially than patients in public hospitals. In this case, the patient in the private hospital seemingly occupies a very high rung in the hierarchy. However, we may also wish to reflect on the degree to which this deference is 'real' or part of a trained 'presentation of self' on the part of the nurses. An example may help to make this clear. Most workers who deal directly with the general public are probably all trained (either formally or informally) in how to deal with and manage their customers. Perhaps, too, staff in private hospitals are trained in a similar, if different, way. We might even ponder on the degree to which *all* nurses should be given such 'people management' training. A criticism, as noted above, is that this is sometimes thought to be insincere, or not 'real'. However, we might counter this by noting that *all* of our communication skills have, at some stage, been learned. Almost all of them, too, arise out of our culture.

Who is the book for?

This book is aimed at diploma and undergraduate nursing students, but it should also be a useful reference source for those working in health care, undertaking higher degrees, and those studying for qualifications in other health care-related disciplines. The aim is, more than anything, to make you think about culture and communication. Although books cannot automatically change practice, it is hoped that by observing and thinking about the ways in which we communicate, from a cultural point of view, we can also begin to change our practice. Thus a reflective and critical attitude is called for in reading the book. You may not agree with everything in it, but we hope you will consider the issues and appreciate *why* you do not agree with them.

What is in the book?

This book starts with a general introduction to culture, through definitions and descriptions. In particular, we discuss what is meant when we refer to the concept of 'culture', how culture is a constantly evolving concept, and the current debate, especially among anthropologists, about the very notion of 'culture' itself. It goes on to discuss culture and interpersonal skills.

Later chapters discuss the ways in which culture can impinge on nursing, and on how we 'learn' culture. One chapter offers an overview of the major world religions; however we feel, personally, about religion, it is one of the issues that underpins almost all cultures at some level. There are chapters on the Thai culture and communication research that will serve as a further 'case study' on how culture affects nursing, and one on cultural pitfalls and problems. There is also another case study on how stress affects student nurses in Brunei - another example of how culture can affect nursing. It is suggested that by exploring other peoples' cultures we can better understand our own. Of course, countries are not 'exotic' to themselves: it is often through visitors from other countries that we learn new things about our own.

What this book is not

This book is not a comparative study, nor a definitive guide to a range of different cultures, although many disparate practical and theoretical examples of cultural issues from around the world are provided. In the book, we often compare and contrast British and Thai cultures, for - as much as anyone can - we (particularly Philip Burnard) know more about these cultures than others. We also see them as being very different from each other, and useful as a means of comparison. We hope that this 'difference' will help to highlight a wide range of cultural differences in nursing practice.

Furthermore, the book is not intended to provide the readers with a convenient 'tick box' guide to how to communicate with those from other cultures, nor does it tell you how to care for people from a range of different cultures. There are already many books and articles on transcultural nursing that can help to inform this process. As we have stated, the main aim of this book is to get you to reflect on your own views about culture, and to explore some of the ways in which culture affects communication. We write as nurse educators and researchers. If we can help you to think about the ways in which culture affects all aspects of your own life, possibly also those of your colleagues and your patients, we will have achieved what we set out to do.

Throughout the book there are boxes containing illustrations of specific points made in the text, and also **Questions for reflection**. There are a number of **Case Studies** in which people from different cultures identify how they feel their culture affects their nursing and health care. It should be noted that each of these represents only one person's point of view. They are not studies from which to generalise, but are intended to illustrate how one nurse, in a different culture, feels about his or her own nursing context.

The book also contains **Practice-based Case Studies** from clinical practice for the reader to consider. The purpose of these is to highlight how cultural issues can affect communication and/or other aspects of nursing practice in multicultural societies such as the UK. All of the research reported in this book has been carried out by the authors and/or their colleagues.

We have tried hard not simply to apply cultural principles to clinical practice. It is easy to slip into cultural stereotyping, and if we carry around in our heads a list of 'what Muslims are like' or 'what North Americans are like', we are likely to be surprised. People - including hospital and community patients - cannot easily be slotted into cultural boxes. Once again, we would emphasise the point of this book: that it is intended to make you think about culture and nursing care.

A note about references

There is a belief among some in nursing that only the most modern references should be used in academic writing (Burnard and Gill, 2007). Although this is often true in the field of cutting-edge research, it is not necessarily true in the fields of such things as theory, communication and culture. There is no logical reason why the most recent theories must be the best or most appropriate. This 'older reference' issue is perhaps most clearly demonstrated in the field of religion. Most religious texts are ancient and are not readily revised (indeed, it is held that the Qu'ran must not be revised and can only be understood in its original Arabic). You will find that we have used a range of modern and older texts to illustrate this book. We have also suggested relevant further reading at the end of each chapter.

We hope you will enjoy reading this book and find it useful both in considering your nursing practice and in writing about culture in essays and assignments. Mixing with people from different cultures can enhance our lives, and it is to be hoped that, in return, we can enhance the lives of others, particularly when we can demonstrate that we know a little of their culture.

Philip Burnard and Paul Gill
Caerphilly and Pontyclun, Wales
May 2008

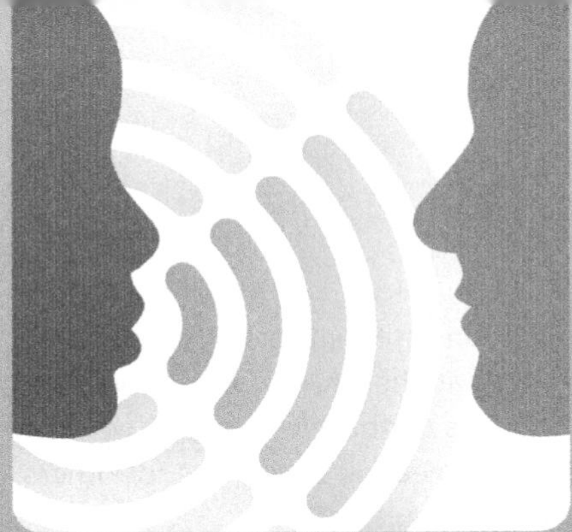

Chapter 1

Thinking about culture

Learning outcomes

At the end of this chapter, you should be able to:

- ✔ define culture
- ✔ relate culture to nursing practice
- ✔ think about how culture defines you, your family, friends, patients and colleagues
- ✔ identify different types of culture

Introduction

This opening chapter first offers some general ways of thinking about culture. It examines different uses of the term, from 'popular culture' to 'anthropological views of culture'. The second half of the chapter identifies more formal definitions of culture, and discusses some of the key issues and debates surrounding the concept of culture.

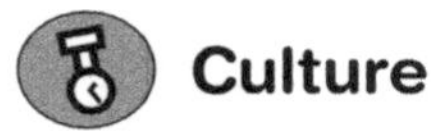

Culture

Culture, and an understanding of it, is an essential part of nursing, particularly in multicultural societies such as the UK. As nurses, we come from a particular cultural background, as do those with whom we work and those we care for. In the process of meeting and caring for others, we come face to face with the meeting of cultures.

The term 'culture' is used the world over. Newspapers report that people coming to the UK should learn about UK culture. There is now even a 'culture test' for those who want to become UK citizens. Politicians, community leaders and sections of the media also emphasise the importance of UK citizens respecting other cultures. In other contexts, phrases such as 'drug culture' or the 'rap culture' may be referred to. But are all of these concepts referred to in the same or similar ways? It might be useful to explore some of the different ways in which the word culture is used. Before that, consider the following:

Question for reflection

How would *you* define the word 'culture'?

The term and the concept of 'culture' are often used in different ways. For example:

High culture This is usually used to refer to the arts - music, painting, sculpture, dance and so on (Gans, 1999). Different styles of art exist in different parts of the world, and what is considered beautiful in one country may not necessarily be viewed that way in others. Sometimes, in history, attempts have been made to censor or direct what may pass as art. In the Stalinist period of Russian communism, for example, composers and painters were encouraged to produce works that appealed to 'the people', and were sometimes condemned for producing work that was considered too highbrow (Gans, 1999). In some languages this is the *only* definition of the word 'culture': in those languages, culture refers only to the arts.

Popular culture This is usually seen as part of academic studies into the everyday and changing patterns of what ordinary people are interested in. Thus a person who studies popular culture might be interested in comics, pop, rock and other sorts of music, fashions, language styles and so on (Collins, 2002). Interestingly, for a discipline that concentrates on the everyday lives of people, the literature that arises out of popular culture studies is often extremely difficult to read because of the complex language chosen by many of those who write in that field.

Subcultures This refers to subsections of any particular society. Thus, in the UK, examples of subcultures may be 'Goths', those who take drugs, those who are very religious (or even those of a particular religious sect). A broader example of subculture (and one that overlaps with popular culture) is the idea of a 'youth subculture', a means of grouping together all young people as likely to be interested in certain things that older or much younger people may not be interested in.

Culture from an anthropological perspective This is the sense in which culture is being discussed in this book. As we shall see from the next section, called 'Formal definitions of culture', the use of 'culture' in this way refers to the ways in which people in a given society live together, and how they communicate with each other (Hendry, 2008). Culture in this sense also refers to how people behave, interact, and live together in a social sense: their religious views (or lack of them) and practices, the ways in which they organise their society, make laws, educate others, even how they talk to each other (Rapport and Overing, 2006). We can, for example, talk about the culture of the UK or the culture of Japan, and in doing so notice some similarities but also some considerable differences. We will probably find that if we visit a culture that is very different from our own, we simply will not always know what is going on. We do not know why people do or say the things that they do.

However, it is important to remember that culture is something we all have: it is not confined to 'other people', and it is certainly not confined to ethnic minority groups, even if their culture appears to be vastly different from our own (which is when we tend to notice 'culture' most). If the cultural beliefs and practices of others seem strange to us, then the converse is also likely to be true, i.e. our own beliefs and practices may seem strange to others. The point to remember here, particularly in a nursing context, is that we are all cultural beings. For example, in a nursing context, we may be surprised at the ways in which patients, doctors or nurses are treated. All of these things happen, perhaps, because we constantly compare other cultures with our own. There is often an expectation among people that others will be like 'us', and of course sometimes they are and sometimes they are not.

One of the key issues in understanding another culture is being able to speak the language of the country in which that culture is located. Language is an important way in which culture is conveyed (Barnard and Spencer, 2002). However, even in countries where the language is the same, the cultural use of that language may lead to misunderstandings. A simple example of this is a comparison of the UK and the US senses of humour. Sometimes, both groups can understand each others' humour. At other times, however, things that people in the US find funny do not seem in the least bit funny in the UK, and vice versa.

Social anthropologists, like psychologists and sociologists, study people, albeit usually in a social context (Hendry, 2008). This will be discussed further later, but it is worth making a few points here. **Anthropology** has changed over many decades. Traditionally, anthropologists tended to be from the West (particularly the UK, France and North America), and primarily conducted research with people from 'exotic', small-scale, non-western societies (Kuper, 1996), which tended to be very different from their own. In conducting such research (described as ethnographic fieldwork), anthropologists would visit a particular country for varying lengths of time – often several years – make notes of their observations and conversations, and then write up an explanation of what was occurring in that society, particularly in relation to human beliefs and behaviours. Because of the frequent differences between the society of the anthropologist and that of the people they were studying, anthropologists were able to take an objective outsider view of that society. This would effectively allow them to compare and contrast beliefs, views and behaviours between the two cultures (Evans-Pritchard, 1962). However, modern social anthropology is now equally concerned with conducting research among people in western societies.

A more recent debate among anthropologists has concerned the appropriateness and ability of a person from outside a culture to enter that culture and really understand it. This has led to accounts of cultures being obtained as a process of negotiation between an 'insider' (i.e. a person who lives within the society being studied) and a **cultural outsider** from another culture (e.g. the anthropologist). Most recently, however, there has been debate about the appropriateness and relevance of the very notion of 'culture' itself (Agar, 2006) - this is discussed further later on in the chapter. There is certainly a danger in thinking that all people in a particular culture will behave in the same or similar ways, and this leads to debate about whether cultural influences are the main things that motivate people (Barnard and Spencer, 2002) or whether other factors, including individual choice, influence human behaviour and can also, perhaps, even override a person's cultural conditioning.

That last point may usefully be elaborated a little. Many children, as they move into adolescence, challenge their parents' views and the cultural norms that those parents, and even their society, live by. When, in turn, those children become adults and have children themselves, they usually find that their offspring also question, in the same sorts of ways. Does this mean that the culture is constantly changing, or that, as individuals grow, they choose to think for themselves? There is probably a middle ground here. Humans are certainly influenced by the culture in which they grow up and live, but we are conscious, thinking beings, who can either go along with society and cultural norms or choose to live differently. We will return to this issue later in this chapter, but first it may be useful to explore other opinions about culture.

Some formal definitions of culture

As already noted, all humans live within and are influenced by culture, yet most of the time our own culture is taken for granted. We usually only notice culture when we see someone else's, particularly if it is different from our own. This chapter explores the notion of culture and relates it to international differences in interpersonal communication.

The term 'culture' is used widely, albeit often inappropriately and, occasionally, incorrectly. Leach (1982) maintains that, over the years, culture as an anthropological concept has undergone many transformations, to the extent that there is now no consensus about how the term should be used. Although many definitions of culture exist, the concept, much like health, is somewhat difficult to define unequivocally. Many people have an idea of what culture is, but would probably find it hard to describe.

Sapir (1948), defines culture as embodying any socially inherited element in the life of man, material and spiritual. In Linton's (1945) terms, the culture of society is the way of life of its members: the collection of ideas and habits which they learn, share and transmit from generation to generation. Harris (1999) asserts that a culture is the socially learned ways of living found in human societies, and that it embraces all aspects of social life, including both thought and behaviour. In the field of nursing, Leininger (1991) provides a more concise definition for the concept of culture as the 'learned, shared and transmitted values, beliefs, norms, and lifeways of a particular group that guides their thinking, decisions, and actions in patterned ways'.

Kluckhohn (1969) offers a breakdown of possible definitions, as follows. First, culture covers the total way of life of a particular set of people. Second, it refers to what individuals acquire from the group they belong to. Third, it is about ways of feeling, thinking and behaving. Fourth, it is an abstract way of looking at behaviour. Fifth, it is anthropological theory (and more will be said about this later). Sixth, it is a collection of pooled learning. Seventh, it is a set of responses to recurrent problems in a particular group. Eighth, it is about learned behaviour. Ninth, it refers to a way of regulating behaviour. Tenth, it is a set of ways for adjusting to the environment and to other people. Eleventh, it is what emerges from history; and twelfth, it is a map of behaviour.

Culture is often described as that which includes knowledge, belief, morals, laws, customs and any other attributes acquired by a person as a member of society (McLaren, 1998). Nemetz Robinson (1985) made the following distinction about definitions of culture: some definitions refer to *culture as observable phenomenon and behaviour*, and some definitions reflect the idea of *culture as not observable* - something that is going on 'under the surface'.

Thus culture may involve observable behaviours but also a felt sense – a sense, perhaps, of identity, of who we are. When we communicate interculturally, we not only communicate words and ideas but also something of ourselves and of our roots.

The value of the study of culture to nursing is fairly clear, and it is a study that is usually undertaken under the umbrella of the discipline of anthropology. Ellsworth (1994) offers a useful summary of some of the reasons why we might apply a study of culture to nursing. She suggests that cultures differ in their definitions of things such as novelty, opportunity, gratification and loss, and in their definition of the right way of responding to these. She also suggests that people vary in the way they view illness: some see it as caused by germs, others by God, chance or witchcraft, or even a person's own moral failure (perhaps caused by 'sin'), and that a person's response to illness will be a reflection of these beliefs. All of these perceptions, when held by different patients in our care, are important. We cannot assume that our patients will hold the same views of illness as we do, nor can we assume that they hold the same views about death.

Culture is also constantly changing and evolving. No society or community is static. Just as language evolves, so do all of the other aspects of culture (Hendry, 2008). Cultures continue to modify themselves in the light of things such as technology, research-based evidence, political change, the financial climate, strife (e.g. conflict) and even fashion. Communication patterns also change in this way.

Clarity and misunderstanding are key issues in **communication.** Those coming to this country, or going to another, have to learn not only a language but also a set of what might be called 'communication rules'. This is often an acute problem for the person coming to work as a student or as a nurse. However, all parties can learn from this anxiety. It is possible to learn a considerable amount about our own communication patterns by observing 'different' ones in students, colleagues or friends coming from another culture and/or society.

How well we communicate depends on how we behave. After language, non-verbal communication seems to be the key factor that enhances or detracts from the way we communicate with others. The behaviours involved in non-verbal communication need to be clear and unambiguous. Further, when we use non-verbal behaviour, we need to be confident that the other person or persons will understand it. So the newcomer to a culture not only has to learn a set of non-verbal behaviours, but also has to learn the 'right' ones to use at any given time.

A familiar problem with anyone entering a different culture is the sudden or gradual realisation of 'difference'. The behaviours and ways of communicating that we take for granted are, suddenly, not those being used around us. This jarring is sometimes termed **culture shock** (Dodd, 1991). Culture shock is the sensation we feel when in a foreign country, where we find that what we expect does not happen, or what we do not expect does happen. This can often cause bewilderment and anxiety, especially in those experiencing it for the first time. What is happening, of course, is that *we* are the foreigner. It is not until we begin to adapt to the way people do things in the country we are visiting that we can begin to relax and allow ourselves to be accepted. Cultures differ in the degree to which they accept outsiders. For example, Mulder (2002), an anthropologist who studied Thai culture for many decades, noted that he would leave that country without having made one close friend. Some countries embrace foreigners, whereas others do not. This should not, however, be confused with **racism.** The countries that do not easily accommodate foreigners are often ones in which dedication to family is important. In those cultures, the person's family and friends (and country) come before all else.

In a 'foreign' culture, one is first of all aware of one's cultural difference rather than one's personal difference. It is I who stand out in the foreign culture. We may, for example, think that most people eat with a knife and fork and feel suddenly out of place when everyone else uses a spoon and fork, or chopsticks. As an extension of this, it is worth noting that 'western' ways of using a knife and fork can also vary. Watch, for example, how many people in the US cut up their food into manageable pieces before putting down the knife and eating with the fork, whereas people in the UK usually use their knives and forks together. Thai people eat with a spoon and fork, except when eating noodles, for which they use chopsticks. For some older Thai people, putting a fork in your mouth amounts to rudeness similar to that registered by some people in the UK who see others putting a knife in their mouths.

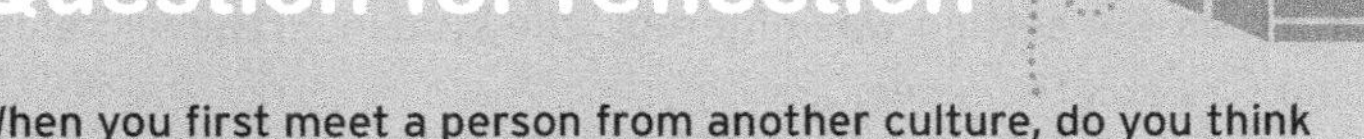

Question for reflection

When you first meet a person from another culture, do you think of them firstly as a *person*, or as *foreign*?

UK nurses might also feed elderly people with a spoon. Many UK patients will probably not be used to eating main courses with a spoon, and the experience might seem very odd. Similarly, drinking from a feeding cup feels strange, and those who have not drunk tea or coffee in this way should at least try it, if only to experience it.

There are huge numbers of cultural variables to be considered when thinking about verbal and non-verbal communication. This book can only consider a few key elements. What follows are some examples of the sort of thing nurses might consider when thinking about cultural aspects of communication. In them, we see the 'taken for granted' questioned by cultural practice.

Case Study

Culture and nursing: a Greek nurse's point of view

My personal experience with cultural differences began with my arrival at the UK university where I began my nursing studies. At that time my Greek background influenced my behaviour and ways of communicating with my university lecturers and professors, my fellow students and my patients.

One simple example was the way the other students casually called their professors by their first name, which was culturally impossible for me. In Greece this would be considered an act of disrespect for a person who has obtained certain credentials and holds such a high position within the community. The professor's word is never questioned, his word is law. In general, persons in respected positions are not referred to by their first names. I felt comfortable when addressing people using Mr, Mrs or Professor. Referring to a teacher by first name made me feel very uncomfortable, since in my culture I had been forbidden to do so. The same

restriction also applied on the ward with my nurse—preceptor: although the setting was different, the student—teacher relationship was still the same.

Another interesting cultural difference was that my fellow students were often on their own, with no financial or emotional support from their parents. This was very strange, since the Greek family is very close and the children are still considered children even in their 60s. I was surprised when most of my fellow students did not want to go back home to be near their parents, but it might be that they were not welcome, as they had been forced out on their own at such an early age. The feeling of being independent is something that Greek children dream about; however, the thought of actually experiencing such a life is very threatening. They know that their Greek family will never allow that to happen. Even in the tragic event of a death in the family, other extended family members take over the role of protecting and nurturing the family. Strange as this cultural difference seems to me, I am sure that people from the UK might consider the Greek family to be too interfering. This is often true, but it is understood that this is usually done with the best intentions and with unconditional love for the child.

My observations were that the UK nurses appeared warmer and kinder than many of the Greek nurses. This could be for many reasons, too many for me to judge without a proper study. A few guesses I would like to offer are that the UK nurses are not permanent employees and could lose their job if they acted in any other way. Other possibilities are that nurses may be looking for the warmth and affection that many do not find in their personal life. Or, of course, they are just kind and caring persons. I would like to believe it is the last, as they would be unlikely to enter into such a difficult position where they are overworked and underpaid unless they genuinely liked helping people.

The Greek nurses, on the other hand, do have a permanent job for life, which unfortunately allows them to sometimes be rude to patients and their families. Most of these nurses come from very loving families and communities, so they do not need to look for warmth and affection from their patients. These same warm families cause distress among nurses, since there are always many family members trying to stay with the patient. It seems unfair that, although the nurses constantly complain about these family members, they do allow one member to stay in order for them to carry out the more personal care which the nurses do not want to offer.

Differences in communication are seen when serious issues occur, such as a diagnosis of cancer. Nurses need to withhold the truth from the patient, and even some family members are not told, such as older people and pregnant women. The stronger family member is told and he determines how much information is passed on to the other family members. I believe this is one of the biggest differences between the two cultures. Usually the patient is not told. I remember one woman, mother of five little children, whose cancer had progressed before it was discovered. The doctors told her husband that she had 3 months to live, but eventually she lived for 6 months. Everyone knew, but no one admitted it to her: she believed her family when they told her that her colostomy was temporary, and that radiation treatment was needed as a precaution, 'just in case'. I am sure other cultures would disagree with this and feel that she should have been told, since she was cheated out of the opportunity of discussing her future death. However, one day I saw her husband try to tell her, but when he saw how frightened and depressed she became, he changed the story back to the 'just in case' scenario.

Most Greek people feel death is certain for all cancer patients, even though this is no longer so. One Greek fellow who had cancer but was unaware of it visited Australia with his wife. There he became ill and was hospitalised. The doctors there refused to abide by his wife's wishes and told him about the cancer. He became very depressed and suffered much more from his fears than before he was told. Another fellow was living in America, where they told him he should leave the hospital and 'go home to die'. Greeks find this behaviour despicable, as they feel that 'hope' is so important to the patient and his family.

Upon my return to Greece, I also faced many cultural dilemmas. Now I had a Master's degree and was working as a staff nurse. I had been trained in the UK and was prepared to offer my nursing skills and knowledge in the Greek setting. Many times when fellow colleagues asked me where I trained I had the impression that they were impressed, yet at the same time intimidated when they heard my answer. Their response indicated that they doubted their abilities in comparison to mine, especially if they had never been abroad. Many felt uncomfortable to provide nursing care in my presence. This was demonstrated when they asked me 'Is this how they do it in the UK?'

In terms of communication with the patients, this was not an issue in the Greek health-care setting. The nurse's role is only to follow doctors' orders, and only in specific settings are support, counselling and rehabilitation offered by nurses, and those settings are very, very limited. On a general ward, the nurse is not expected to build a rapport with the patient. This situation put me in another cultural predicament. Instinctively from my training I was always trying to communicate with the patients and their families. Unfortunately, the response of my fellow nurses was not as I had expected. Some, I like to think, were positively influenced; others used the excuse that I am young, and that in a few years I too will become like them and not respond so warmly to the patients and their relatives. At that point I needed to make a decision. It was impossible for me, from the position of staff nurse, and having trained abroad, to implement a change, and so I had to decide whether I wanted to become like my fellow nurses, so I could fit in with them, or to offer the nursing care in the way that I had been trained to do. Finally, I decided that I could not disregard all my years of study: I felt compelled to offer the nursing care I knew, with my strengths and weaknesses, in the best interests of my patients. Once my decision was made and I was willing to deal with the consequences, I became aware of other nurses responding to my behaviour. Some seemed to admire my actions: a few even claimed that they were learning from me, whereas others offered strange looks and were waiting for me to grow out of it.

Of course the attitude of the last group gave me even more strength to keep up my communication skills with my patients. As it was a university hospital, a teaching institute, I had some Greek student nurses who followed me while I carried out my duties. I was surprised when they complained about how disgusted they were with those nurses' attitudes, illustrating that newer nurses were aware of the importance of implementing communication skills in their nursing care.

In Greece, in general, there has been a great disrespect and lack of trust towards the nursing profession. Many people are not even aware that nursing is a university degree course and considered a science. Now, slowly, these better-educated nurses are taking up positions in nursing, and hopefully a higher standard of care will be offered, with a more holistic approach.

Question for reflection

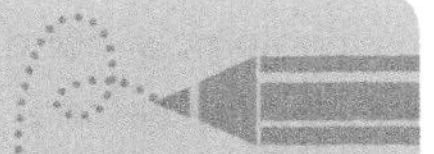

What, in your view, are the biggest differences between this Greek nurse's experience and yours?

Individualist and collectivist cultures

The distinction has been made between **individualist societies,** in which 'I' comes before 'we', and **collectivist societies** in which 'we' comes before 'I' (McLaren, 1998). Hofstede (1994) describes these differences as follows: individualist societies are those in which ties between individuals are loose and most people are expected to look after themselves. In collectivist societies, people are born into families with a strong sense of collective identity and responsibility for one another. In other words, in the collectivist society the family is often more important than any single member of it.

It may be hypothesised, then, that students from an individualist culture, with its emphasis on values such as self-motivation and self-development, may express higher levels of self-esteem than students from collectivist cultures in which emphases are on values such as working together, respect for others and the fulfilment of others' needs (Triandis, 1972).

Hofstede (1994) suggests that the vast majority of people in the world live in collectivist societies, in which the interest of the group prevails over the interest of the individual. The first group, in the collectivist society, is the family into which a person is born. In most collectivist societies, the 'family' within which the child grows up consists of people living closely together, not just the parents and other children, but also grandparents, aunts, servants or other housemates - the extended family. When children grow up they learn to consider themselves as part of the *we* group, a relationship that is not voluntary but given. The *we* group is usually distinct from other people in society, who belong to a *they* group, of which there are many. The *we* group is the major source of identity for the person in a collectivist culture, and often the only security they have against the hardships of life. A strong practical and psychological bond forms between the person and the *we* group to which they belong.

However, as Triandis *et al.* (1991) note, we need to be cautious about such distinctions and use them perhaps as a general guide: it is not sufficient merely to know about the culture from which a person comes; we also need to consider issues such as movement from country settings to town settings, affluent settings as opposed to poor ones, travel and immigration (e.g. to and from other countries), and also the degree to which people are exposed to the media. It is notable that in urban cultures there is often a far greater 'smoothing out' and internationalisation of culture.

Hofstede (1994) also noted that almost everyone belongs to a range of different groups and categories at the same time. He offers the following examples:

- A national level according to one's country (or countries, for people who migrated during their lifetime);
- A regional and/or ethnic and/or religious and/or linguistic affiliation level, as most nations are composed of culturally different regions and/or ethnic and/or religious and/or language groups;

- A gender level, according to whether a person was born as a girl or as a boy;
- A social class level, which separates grandparents from parents and children;
- For those who are employed, an organisational or corporate level according to the way employees have been socialised by their work organisation (Hofstede, 1994).

Perhaps, however, the notions of 'individuality' and of 'the individual' are beginning to wane, in some countries at least. Frie (2003) notes the impact of postmodernity on the self and the individual:

> ***In contrast to the modernist emphasis on the autonomy of the individual mind, postmodernism asserts that the person, or subject, is not only shaped but also subverted by the contexts in which it exists. More radical versions of postmodernism deny the very existence of a person with the capacity for reflexive thought and self-determining action. In place of the person as an active, responsible being, they herald the so-called death of the subject.***
>
> ***(Frie, 2003)***

Post-modernists usually claim that the world around us is something of a construct. We do not 'discover reality' but invent it (Watzlawick, 1984). We cannot apprehend the world directly or objectively, but only through language and the notions and concepts we have invented. We are not able to measure our thoughts against any objective reality as we cannot transcend or stand outside our own concepts or language. It is impossible, then, for us to achieve any sort of undistorted view of the world (Frederickson, 2003). All of this applies equally to our attempting to understand other cultures and other peoples. We have no way of knowing that what we are observing reflects any sort of verifiable 'truth'. Just as the post-modernists suggest that 'the reader writes the text', so we might say that the cultural observer or ethnographer 'invents the culture' that he or she observes from their own subjective viewpoint.

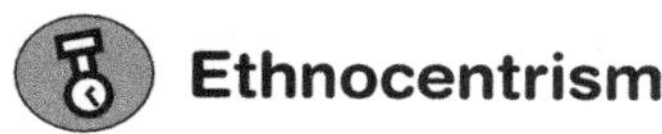

Ethnocentrism

Ethnocentrism is essentially the belief in the inherent superiority of one's own cultural group (Van Der Geest, 1995). The idea of ethnocentrism, however, is thought to have started with the sociologist William Sumner (1906). He suggested that it was the name we gave to a view of things in which our own group is the centre of everything, and that all other groups are measured against our own.

Question for reflection

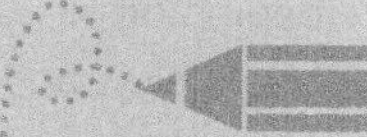

To what degree do you see your own country as being 'right' in the way it does things and to what degree do you make comparisons between your own 'right' way of doing things and the way things are done in other countries? This is something of a measure of our own tendency towards ethnocentrism.

Such a position is inevitable: as we have noted, we are all bound by our own culture and our immersion and upbringing within it. Research has supported the idea that similarity of culture will be a determining factor in our attitude towards others. Wanguri (1996) notes that we tend to like people who are similar to us and dislike those who are dissimilar to us. This is perhaps too strong a position. We are, after all, often attracted also to the 'difference' in other people. The point is, perhaps, that ethnocentrism becomes a problem when we are unconscious of it. Hellweg *et al.* (1991) make the following point: ethnocentricity is often invisible (for example, those who are Western often almost 'naturally' assume that a Western way of doing things is right and measure all other cultures against it). And of course, other cultures look out from their countries and view other 'foreigners' in the same way.

It is almost as if we all live with a large group of others in huge, invisible castles from which we look out and make judgements about other people's ways of life. This has become very noticeable in recent years, where Islamic commentators have viewed Western ways of doing things and North Americans have viewed Muslims in the same sort of way. Both have a strong tendency to see their particular way of doing things as 'right' and the other group as necessarily being 'wrong', or 'less right'.

Question for reflection

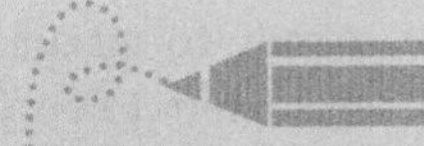

To what degree do you feel this *book* is ethnocentric? It may be impossible for anyone to escape the trap of ethnocentricity. Would you consider yourself to be ethnocentric?

The concept of ethnocentrism is further compounded by the ways in which society views expressions of it. Describing this 'tangle', Korzenny (1991) suggests that we are mostly likely to be positive about those who are similar to us, but also suggests that we can convincingly deny this both to ourselves and to our colleagues. He suggests that denial of ethnocentrism is one of the most powerful barriers to intercultural communication, because that denial prevents confrontation, clarification and acceptance of others.

Practice-based Case Study

Brain death in a Japanese tourist

In the mid-1990s I was working as a senior staff nurse in a regional intensive therapy unit (ITU) in a major UK city. One evening we had a patient admitted to the unit who had been involved, as a pedestrian, in a road traffic accident. The man was in his mid-forties and was a Japanese tourist, visiting the UK on a sightseeing holiday with his family. The family spoke reasonable English, although the son and daughter (both teenagers) spoke very good English.

The man had sustained a serious head injury, which included a depressed skull fracture and a large subdural haematoma (brain haemorrhage) that required neurosurgery. Despite surgical intervention, Akira* (*a pseudonym) never regained consciousness, and after several days on a ventilator it became clear that his brain injury had worsened significantly, to the extent that he met the criteria for brainstem death testing.

At this stage Akira was tested for brainstem death and it was subsequently confirmed that he was brainstem dead. As Akira also met the criteria to become a multiorgan donor, if his family consented, a consultant anaesthetist and I initially approached the family to discuss the results of the brainstem death tests and to ask them to consider this option.

However, significant problems arose when we tried to communicate this to the family. Brainstem death is often a difficult concept for families in ITU to understand, primarily because of the circumstances, and especially because the patient is often warm and still has a heartbeat. However, the family rejected the prospect of organ donation out of hand and were extremely vociferous in their refusal to accept that Akira was really dead while his heart was still beating.

At first, the medical team all felt that this situation was probably due to language issues. No one really considered that it might in fact be due to social and cultural factors. Consequently, the medical team decided to involve a Japanese senior house officer in anaesthetics to help explain the situation to the family. It was only at this stage that it became clear that the reason they did not accept brain death as a 'proper definition of death' was because of their cultural background. The Japanese doctor, along with Akira's eldest son, subsequently explained to us that the family (apparently as with many Japanese people) believed that the body and the spirit were mutually connected and that the *kokora* (a very old metaphorical concept that represents a region, probably in the thorax, where the human spirit or soul resides), not the brain, represented the 'humane part of the person' (Gill, 2000). Therefore, while Akira still had a heartbeat his soul still resided in his body, and hence he was not yet 'really dead'.

Although none of us laughed at or derided the family (even in private) for holding these views, we all felt that they were naïve, illogical and antiquated, primarily because they conflicted with reliable physiological evidence. We simply did not believe that social and cultural issues were as important as biological ones. Although we never forced our beliefs upon the family, we never accepted theirs, although of course we did try to respect them. However, a short time after this incident, Akira's ventilatory support was withdrawn and within a few minutes he 'died' in the traditional sense (i.e. loss of breathing and heartbeat).

It really was only some time afterwards – I suppose when the 'dust had settled' – that I was able to look back on this incident and realise that even though we spoke to the family, we did not really listen to what they had to say. We felt that our beliefs were superior to theirs, as we believed that our reliable, scientific, yet novel notion of brain death was apparently infallible. We could not accept that others held different views, because they seemed outdated and were based on social and cultural issues and therefore, could not be supported by medical evidence.

This incident did, however, teach me a valuable lesson. It highlighted to me that, as a nurse, I needed to respect the beliefs of people from other cultures, whenever possible, even if at times they seemed illogical.

People may attempt to show their lack of ethnocentricity by denying difference and by proclaiming that 'we are all the same under the skin', in a similar way to those who would hold that 'all religions have some truth in them'. The blandishments do little to help us understand both the similarities and the differences of people in other cultures. Although most people have a similar physiological make-up (although differences exist there too), the way our culture shapes us does make us different, to varying degrees, from those who live in other cultures. A useful meeting point between the extremes of 'we are all different' and 'we are all the same', lies with the often-quoted triplet: people are, in certain respects:

- Like *no* other persons
- Like *some* other persons
- Like *all* other persons.

If these points are considered in reverse, it is possible to see that we all have anxieties and worries, all fall in love (or have a similar experience) and all have friends. We are like some other people in being nurses, in being male or female, or in having a particular skin colour. Finally, we are like no other people in being 'ourselves'. This is probably, by definition, the most difficult area in which to give examples.

What this triplet shows is that we are not really unique. There has been a temptation in nursing over the past few decades to declare that 'everyone is unique', and this has led to a drive towards 'patient-centred' care or 'individualised care'. Probably neither is economically or practically possible. Everyone has unique features, but it is an over-statement to say that each of us is a 'one-off' and unique. Although we do have aspects that are personal to us, we also share many aspects with huge numbers of others. People are, after all, sociable beings. We do not live in complete isolation, unless we choose to. The fact that many people usually enjoy being with others, even if not all of the time, may militate against the notions of patient-centred and individualised care. Perhaps, sometimes we all enjoy being part of the crowd.

However, a more complicated thought about the above triplet is that it is not difficult to say in what ways we are similar to all other people (we all have to eat and drink, for example). Neither is it difficult to say in what ways we are similar to some others (we generally know that we are male or female, what our political views are, that we are nurses, etc.). But how do we conceptualise and discuss the ways in which we are like *no* other people? What sort of language would be required to convey to another person the ways in which we are unique? Perhaps, theoretically speaking, if we really were unique, it seems likely that the listener would not understand what we were saying, because, by definition, it would be outside their experience.

Question for reflection

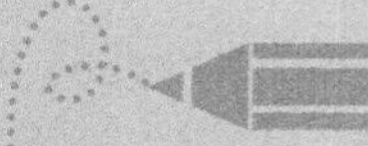

Can you think of three ways in which you are 'like no other person'?

Writing of the difficulties of facing both our own ethnocentrism and our own ignorance of other cultures, Said (1979) states:

For if it is true that no production of knowledge in the human sciences can ever ignore or disclaim its author's involvement as a human subject in his own circumstances, then it must also be true that for a European or North

American studying the Orient, there can be no disclaiming the main circumstances of his actuality: that he comes up against the Orient as a European or American first, as an individual second. *(Said, 1979)*

It seems reasonable to claim that the perceptive visitor has a clearer and newer view of what he or she is seeing and experiencing. He or she 'sees' things in another culture that the resident has grown familiar with to the point of filtering it out of his or her sensory perception mechanisms. Keeping that 'freshness' may be an important factor in working at the development of **ethnography.**

It is important not to get carried away by the concept of culture, though, because it is generally acknowledged that culture is only one of a number of factors that impinge on and influence people's lives. Writing on factors that affect health, Helman (2001) comments that:

. . . the culture into which you are born, or in which you live, is by no means the only such influence. It is only one of a number of influences, which includes individual factors (such as age, gender, size, appearance, personality, intelligence and experience), educational factors (both formal and informal and including education into a religious, ethnic or professional subculture), and socioeconomic factors (such as social class, economic status, and the networks of social support from other people). *(Helman, 2001)*

Indeed, it could be argued that so many factors influence both us as individuals and society as a whole, that it is often difficult to disentangle everything in order to establish 'what does what'.

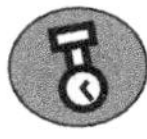

Face

The expression 'to save face' is common in the UK, but **face** is not such an important issue in this country as in many Eastern ones. Face is about maintaining dignity, of not being made to look foolish and of retaining status. In countries where face is an important concept, for example, teachers will work hard to maintain their students' face by not embarrassing them. Students will almost *never* put a teacher in a position of losing face, for to make a teacher lose face is also to lose face oneself. Many lecturers in UK schools and colleges of nursing, sometimes ponder on how to make students from Eastern countries participate more in discussions. Many such students will not do so for at least the following four reasons:

1. They cannot keep up with the discussion, because of language differences.
2. They do not want to risk disagreeing with the lecturer, for if the student is right in his or her disagreement, the lecturer will lose face.
3. If the lecturer loses face, so will the student.
4. The student will be keen to 'get the answer right'. Although UK lecturers may insist that, in discussions, there are no right answers, the student may well feel she or he has lost face if they think they have got an answer wrong.

Giving 'wrong' answers and losing face may lead to various confusions. In a number of cultures, such as Japanese and Thai, it is often considered rude to say 'no' to people. This leads to vague responses to questions where the answer in the UK would be 'no'. In some cultures, too, the 'no' response will not be forthcoming at all. It is widely advised in travel books not to ask of a local, 'Is the temple this way?', for the answer will invariably be 'yes', to save face for both the visitor and the one giving the information. A better question would be: 'Is the temple *this* way or *that* way?' This means that the listener can give a positive direction and not run the risk of having to correct the inquirer and thus risk loss of face.

Face also extends to the clinical setting. When undertaking nursing procedures for patients from cultures where face is important, nurses should be careful not to expose the body too much, and should take care not to embarrass the patient in other ways. Face is an enduring concept, and 'lost' or 'broken' face can be a source of very severe humiliation.

Face also accounts, to some degree, for why patients from Eastern countries will often seek opinions from doctors rather than nurses.

Doctors have higher status in those patients' eyes, and a) are therefore more likely to be accurate in their answers, and b) should not be subjected to the risk of losing face by having the patient seek advice from a more junior member of staff.

In a country such as the UK, where there is something of a 'flattened hierarchy' and status and face do not count for so much, it is easy to be dismissive of it when it occurs in those from other cultures, but, as discussed above, face is a hugely important concept in many cultures and not one to be dismissed lightly.

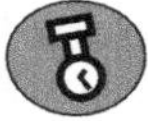

Value sets

Who and what we value often informs our cultural identity. In the West, the ordering of our allegiance values is often like this:

- Me and my immediate family
- My friends
- My work colleagues
- Eventually, my community and my country.

In Eastern cultures, however, the ordering of allegiance values is often as follows:

- The monarch and the country
- My immediate family
- Me
- My friends
- Other people.

Such ordering will make a significant difference to the way in which we interact with others, particularly those outside our immediate family. In the UK, as already noted, we tend towards individualism - the idea that 'I' am important, and that I need to take care of myself. In other cultures, however, it is very common for a person to value his family and friends before himself.

Nationalism

Nationalism, simply put, is the idea of needing to have a particular allegiance to the nation in which we were born and/or raised. It can be argued, from this point of view, that birth determines nationality, although of course it is also possible to choose to change nationality. For example, if a person was born in one country but lived in another for most of their life, they may feel a stronger allegiance to the country in which they now reside.

Nationalism can work in several opposing ways. In times of war, it can help an invaded country to close ranks and become determined to ward off oppressors, almost acting as a single body: 'the nation'. The other side of this is that, again in war, it can lead to oppressing countries believing that they have a natural superiority over those whom they invade. It is possible to look around the world and see both positive and negative aspects of nationalism at work.

Racism

Racism is perhaps an extreme form of nationalism. It is where one country, one culture or one race sees itself as superior to all others. To this end, depending on the strength of feeling, nations or individuals who are racist may take direct, aggressive action against those who are outside their own group.

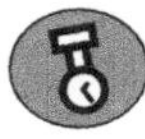

Is there such a thing as culture?

Despite all the definitions and the discussion, there remains a popular debate, particularly among anthropologists, about whether there is such a thing as 'culture'. Michael Agar, a well-known anthropologist, questions the notion of culture:

The culture concept is a mess in anthropology. Where did such a nice concept go wrong? In the old days, we used to describe, to explain, and to generalise. A person did

something, so it was their culture. Why did they do it? Because it was their culture. Who were they? They were members of that culture.

It just doesn't work like that anymore. It may never have, but we pretended that it did. *(Agar, 2006)*

Like many anthropologists, Agar (2006) is particularly critical of the idea that cultures are somehow 'set in stone', or closed systems that rarely, if ever, change. He also suggests that, increasingly, most people are part of a variety of cultures. For example, in Brixton, south London, it is not uncommon to hear young white English people, born in the country, using a Caribbean accent and using 'gangsta rap' hand gestures in communicating with their friends. It is possible that the accent and some of the gestures are dropped when they are at school or college. Similarly, it is possible to hear young black people, born in the UK, adopting both the Caribbean accent and the hand gestures. What is the predominant culture here? English? Caribbean? Afro-American? Agar suggests that we might be more accurate in referring to 'cultures' rather than 'culture'. Again, we can see that we are all perhaps a mixture of different cultures, particularly in the West and increasingly in the East.

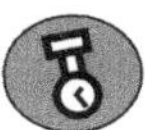

Cultural sensitivity

Cultural sensitivity is a concept related to ethnocentrism and culture shock. It is the ability to appreciate that, although it may not be possible to fully understand another culture, it is possible to understand at least some aspects of it (Barnard and Spencer, 2002). Hanvey (1979) identifies four stages in this process:

1. The stage of stereotypes, of awareness of superficial or very visible cultural traits. This limited awareness usually comes from brief travel and from reading popular magazines. The differences noted seem exotic and bizarre.
2. The stage when a person notices unfamiliar significant and subtle cultural traits. This often comes from cultural conflict situations and seems frustrating and irrational.

3. The stage when a person notices unfamiliar significant and subtle cultural traits but analyses them intellectually, accepting them and trying to understand them.
4. Finally, the stage where the person is aware what it is like to belong to another culture. This comes from cultural immersion, from living in the culture. The person not only understands, as in stage 3, but personally empathises with the culture (Hanvey, 1979).

Despite this, the ability to truly stand outside one's own culture and 'be' as a person in another culture, is, arguably, extremely difficult. The first author, despite many visits and stays in Thailand, 8 years later often finds himself suddenly aware that his real understanding of Thailand is minimal. We always take ourselves, perhaps unknowingly, with us. Ultimately, we probably cannot act at all, except out of the culture from which we derive. In Thailand, the sudden silence, the enigmatic smile, the look of surprise, can all indicate that the actor has suddenly transgressed a cultural norm and made the assumption – which surely everyone makes – that 'everyone, at some level, is like me'.

Some people fear the homogeneity of cultures: the concern that, probably led by the United States of America, all cultures are becoming one. Hamelink (cited in Tomlinson, 2000) refers to this 'cultural synchronization' – the process whereby cultural products go only in one direction, damaging the variety of systems worldwide. Although evidence of the effects of Western popular culture and capitalism are to be seen everywhere in Bangkok and other large cities, so is evidence of the sustaining 'difference' of Thai culture. Nor is the movement of change between cultures only from east to west. For example, Asian cultures also affect each other, leading to other worries about the effects of nearer cultures on the home:

> ***The Pakistani government fears the potential of Indian cinema; the Korean and Taiwanese comics industries object to the encroachment of Japanese* manga*; and the Laotian intellectuals resent the influence of Thai popular culture, particularly television, on Lao literature.*** ***(Lent, 1995)***

It seems that, in the end, there probably never was a truly 'pure' culture. Presumably, all countries, from their foundation, have, at various times taken on some of their neighbours' beliefs, behaviours and attitudes?

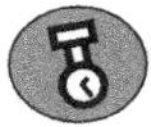

Culture and nursing

The study of culture has most often been associated with the discipline of anthropology, largely because of the people and the societies that anthropologists have traditionally studied. In recent decades, the literature has illustrated the links between anthropology, culture and nursing, often under the heading of 'transcultural nursing'.

Of particular note, in the linkage between anthropology, nursing and culture is the work of Leininger (see, for example, 1991) and the reader is directed to her work for more details of this approach to transcultural nursing. Gerrish (1997) is critical of the notion of transcultural nursing, claiming that it may encourage ethnocentricity by not acknowledging variations in culture within a culture, and variations between generations within a culture. Any attempt to 'capture' a culture seems doomed: there will always be exceptions and cultural variations in all societies.

Gerrish and Papadopoulos (1999) note that Leininger's approach to transcultural nursing adopts a culturalist perspective whereby the aim is for nurses to develop expertise in caring for people from specific ethnic groups. They note that this approach has been strongly criticised for its apparent neglect of racism and of the structural forces that have an impact on the health experiences of ethnic communities (see, for example, Bruni, 1988, Swendson and Windsor, 1996). Indeed, some of Leininger's own writing appears to encourage a form of cultural separatism in nursing. In her 1991 publication, for example, she claims that there may be much merit in care being provided by nurses from the patient's own cultural group.

At the time of writing, and because of a worldwide shortage of nurses, many Western countries are now recruiting nurses from South-east Asia, sometimes to the point of almost decimating the health-care services in those countries. Today, the idea – even if it were acceptable – of patients from a particular culture being cared for by nurses from that culture, seems highly impractical and unlikely.

The issue of cultural integration is complex. Whereas on the surface it would seem preferable to encourage those of different cultures, living in a given society, to integrate freely and for the community to absorb some of their cultural mores, in practice, many people from many cultures prefer to maintain their cultural 'difference'. However, it also seems likely that cultural non-integration might be encouraged by having ethnic 'experts' who, like everyone else, will have their own particular view on the culture they represent.

'Culture', then, is multifaceted and complex. It is neither static nor easily bounded, defined and described. For every 'cultural rule' there would seem to be exceptions, and an attempt to pinpoint a given moment in culture therefore seems problematic. At best, perhaps, anthropologists offer a slightly subjective (and sometimes perhaps even fictional) 'snapshot' of what a culture appeared to be like to them, viewed through a particular lens at a particular point in time. The ethnography that truly illuminates a given cultural setting has probably yet to be written and, for the reasons discussed above, probably never will be: even if it were possible to construct such a monograph, for how long would it be appropriate and relevant?

Conclusion

This chapter started by identifying different meanings of the term 'culture'. It then directed the reader towards the idea of 'anthropological culture' and offered some formal definitions from other writers and researchers in the field. Finally, it explored some of the things that anthropologists think about when considering culture, including the idea that culture itself may nowadays be a less useful term than it once was thought to be. However, it does seem almost self-evident that groups of people, living in different countries and in different parts of those countries, do act, communicate and live in 'different' sorts of ways. Understanding some of those differences, particularly in the area of communication, can be a very fruitful form of study for nurses. The next two chapters explore the ideas of communication and of communication in nursing.

Suggested reading

Andrews MM, Boyle JS (2007). *Transcultural Concepts in Nursing Care*, 5th edn. Baltimore: Lippincott, Williams & Wilkins.

Hendry J (2008). *An Introduction to Social Anthropology: Sharing Our Worlds*, 2nd edn. Basingstoke: Palgrave Macmillan.

Papadopoulos I (2006). *Transcultural Health and Social Care: Development of Culturally Competent Practitioners*. Oxford: Churchill Livingstone.

Rapport N, Overing J (2006). *Social and Cultural Anthropology: the Key Concepts*. London: Routledge.

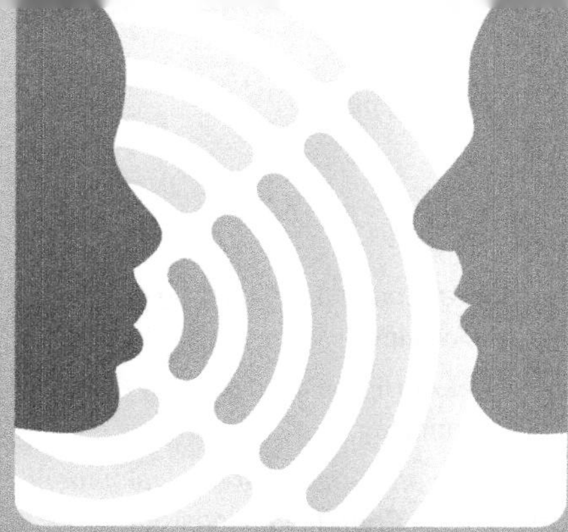

Chapter 2

Communication, nursing and culture

Learning outcomes

At the end of this chapter, you should be able to:

- ✔ identify different types of communication
- ✔ discuss communication in nursing
- ✔ identify problems in health-care communication
- ✔ appreciate some cultural difference in communication

Introduction

This chapter explores the concept of communication among and between people, focusing on key aspects of verbal and non-verbal communication. In particular, cultural variations in communication patterns are explored, along with some potential implications for nursing practice.

What is communication?

We communicate all the time: in fact, we cannot *not* communicate. There is a common tendency to think of communication in terms of speech, conversation, written documents and so on. Or we think of non-verbal communication, which is about the ways in which we use **eye contact**, gestures, **touch** etc. However, we also communicate in numerous other ways, such as the clothes we wear, the symbols we adopt (e.g. the Christian who wears a cross around their neck, or the Buddhist who wears wrist threads), our accents and the use of speech. All of these things, and many more, help to convey messages to other people about who we are. In nursing, all of these aspects of communication come into play, but these aspects of communication may be 'read' differently by patients and nurses from other cultures. There is probably no such thing as 'culture-free' communication.

It will be useful to consider the cultural implications of both verbal and non-verbal aspects of communications, under the following headings:

- Communication hierarchies
- Saying hello and goodbye
- Please and thank you
- **Phatic communication**
- **Listening**, turn-taking and pacing
- **Proximity**
- Touch
- Eye contact
- Volume and **gesture**

Communication hierarchies

In the west, particularly in northern Europe and the USA, people work and communicate together in fairly informal ways. There is what may be called a 'flattened hierarchy' in many organisations. This is still not completely true in the health-care professions, where medical staff tend to view themselves as 'senior' in relation to nursing staff. However, it is increasingly common to use first names, instead of titles and surnames ('Jane', as opposed to 'Dr Hartman') in working situations. Almost paradoxically, though, we should not assume that patients automatically want to be called by their first names, particularly if they are older or have held posts of seniority.

Given the relative lack of hierarchy in western society tends to mean that people can talk fairly freely between themselves, and patients are increasingly questioning and challenging health-care professionals. They are also becoming increasingly knowledgeable about the conditions from which they suffer, partly from television programmes, from reading, and to quite a large degree because of the amount of information available on the internet. Health professionals seem to have mixed views on this. Some see it as an empowering process for the patient, and others (perhaps rightly) are concerned about the status (and possibly the reliability) of the information available on the internet. Whatever the views held by individuals, it seems unlikely that the tide will turn back to a time in which Western patients meekly accepted advice from their doctors and nurses.

The other side to this 'knowledgeable patient' situation is that doctors and other health-care professionals are being increasingly influenced by the notion of evidence-based practice and patient-centred care. Evidence-based practice is concerned with health professionals identifying, through the research literature, the efficiency and effectiveness of particular treatment regimens (Gill, 2004). Clinical judgement is increasingly being supported by all the available research to provide the best possible line of treatment and care. At the same time, health-care practice is increasingly being run along business lines and patients are, to a much greater extent, being viewed as 'customers' or 'clients', with the right to request or challenge the available treatment. The pull, in both directions, in the west, is thus towards a further flattening of the health-care hierarchy.

In the east, however, the notion of a highly structured social hierarchy is much in evidence. In Thailand, for example, no-one is equal to anyone else, and Thai people are adept at quickly identifying where they stand in relation to those with whom they come in contact. Even twins are not equal: the first born is 'senior' to the second born, and the second born will defer to the elder twin. Seniority may be broadly identified in terms of age, education, job and salary. In health-care settings, patients listen to doctors and, to a lesser degree, nurses, and never challenge the advice they are given. They may also be nervous about asking doctors questions if they do not understand a particular plan of treatment, and it often falls to the nurse to act as intermediary or go-between, in the doctor–patient relationship. However, this takes some courage on the nurse's part, as he or she may also be nervous of questioning the doctor.

In Eastern countries, too, professional titles are important and are often used, although in Thailand people are generally known by their first name with a title attached in front. Thus people may be called the equivalent of Dr John or Miss Jane. Even the Thai phonebook is printed in first-name order, rather than by surname.

Except among friends, in the east the normal practice is for senior people to speak first and for junior people to listen and answer questions asked of them. In this sense, eastern cultures often appear very 'polite' in comparison with their western counterparts.

Saying hello and goodbye

People in the UK say hello or hi very frequently during the course of the day, sometimes even extending to saying hello to a colleague each time they meet. In contrast, in a number of Asian cultures, neither hello nor goodbye is frequently used: it is acknowledged that you are there by your presence, and it is not felt necessary to say hello. Similarly, it is fairly obvious when you are leaving and it is not felt necessary to say goodbye. The term for both hello and goodbye, in Thai, is *sawatdee*, and it came into the language only in the 1930s. It is not used frequently among Thais themselves, but is sometimes used to greet foreigners. Departures in Asia can appear abrupt to those from the West, where, particularly in the UK, departures can be very prolonged. Consider the following situation:

Friends have been to your house for a meal and begin to indicate that they will be leaving soon. This will often be heralded by a vague statement, such as 'We must be

thinking about going soon'. Some time later, movements towards leaving will be made, including the collection of coats and perhaps a lengthy discussion about future meetings and meals. You and your friends then stand at the door to make further goodbyes, and you may watch them get into their car. If the car has to be reversed or turned around, the friends may afterwards wind down the window and make further and final goodbyes. The whole process can take some time (anything up to an hour or more) from the initial statement of intent to leave.

Contrast this with a meal in a Chinese house, where, as soon as the meal is finished, guests will usually get up and leave immediately. Similarly, in heath-care settings Asian patients may not expect you to greet them, whereas UK patients may feel affronted if you do not say good morning or good afternoon when you come on duty, or visit them in their houses.

Case Study

Culture and nursing: a Thai nurse's perspective

In Thailand there is a culture of respect towards people who are older than you. In general, the more senior you are, the more respectfully you will be received, particularly by older people. Even though you do something wrong, people are ready to forgive you because you are older, more senior, and have more experience. As an old person you are supported, not blamed.

In nursing practice, this culture of respect has been adopted in how nurses approach patients from different age groups. The interpersonal relationship can be initiated by how we relate to other people. Thus, you could show your respect to older patients by calling them 'father', 'mother', 'grandmother', 'grandfather', 'uncle' etc. This is more common than using a patient's name. The more precise initial name you give needs to be related to your own age. For example, when you are around 20–30 years of age you may need to call patients who are 50 years old 'father' or 'mother'.

Most patients seem to feel happier when they see you are paying respect; they feel more comfortable in the situation and have a lot of self-esteem while being a patient.

However, this practice needs to be validated if you work in a big city, where they are more prone to westernisation and people are more individual. When you call a patient father or mother, he or she may reply that 'I have only child' or 'I'm not your mother': this means that you are not their child, and so you are not supposed to call them father or mother. The interpersonal relationship between patient and nurse in a big city is much more formal and quite distant. Money is power, too, if you are hired as a personal nurse for patients who are better off, to take care of them in their private hospital room. Basically, we do not mind if we provide whatever patients need when they cannot do it for themselves, but sometimes their family may view a personal nurse as a servant or housekeeper, who should provide extensive services to the patient's family as well as their visitors. For example, they may expect the personal nurse to prepare drinks and snacks for the patient's guests, or to turn the TV on and off as the patient or their family request. From time to time it has been brought into discussion in nursing meetings whether these are professional nursing jobs. It was concluded that nurses need to work strictly on their professional jobs and leave the rest to patients' families or housekeepers. This response, of course, does not please the patient's family, who has more of an expectation and has the attitude that they have already paid for a personal nurse, so they must work as a personal assistant too.

In conclusion, providing nursing care in Thailand involves not only the need to bring cultural influences into account, but also cultural changes are needed to keep nursing professional.

Please and thank you

As with hello and goodbye, the saying of please and thank you varies greatly from culture to culture. People in the UK tend to use these words excessively. For example, a conversation in a local newsagent, involving a man buying a newspaper and the woman operating the till, might proceed thus:

> **'Hi. Thanks.' (Man places paper on the counter)**
> **'Thanks. That's 80p please.' (Assistant)**
> **'Thanks.' (Man, searching for money and then giving the money to the assistant)**
> **'Thanks.' (Assistant taking money)**
> **'Thanks.' (Man receiving change)**
> **'Thank you.' (assistant)**
> **'Thanks.' (Man, leaving area)**

This transaction involves seven 'thank yous' in order to buy a single newspaper. In South-east Asia, and probably in many other parts of the world, the transaction might have taken place in silence. The problem with growing up and living in a country where please and thank you are said so frequently is that people from that country tend to perceive those from other cultures, where the words are less frequently said (if at all), as rude. Nurses in the UK are likely to expect patients to thank them for carrying out a particular nursing task, but if the patient comes from another culture such a statement might be deemed unnecessary; it should not, however, be construed as rude.

The other 'automatic' word for many UK people is 'sorry'. If two people bump into each other, it does not matter who was at fault, as both are likely to say 'sorry'. And many people will say 'sorry' when such an apology is not required at all (e.g. 'I'm sorry, but do you have a book on pain care, please?') Again, such automatic responses are not the case in many cultures. Indeed, in Thailand the overuse of please, thank you and sorry is deemed not only to be unnecessary, but even slightly rude itself. If you are working with people from countries that do not use these words very much (or if you are visiting or working in those countries), you would do well to cut down on their usage. For further details about UK manners and customs, see Fox (2005).

This leads to the phrase that often comes up in cultural debates: the idea that 'When in Rome, do as the Romans do'. We sometimes expect that a) people will know the culture they visit, and b) will live their lives according to the norms of that culture. The problems here should be immediately obvious. First, the visitor to another culture cannot be expected to know all about the culture in 'Rome'. Second, we are socialised into our own culture at a very early point in our lives, and breaking our own norms may be very difficult. Just try, for example, not to say sorry next time someone bumps into you, or not to say thank you when buying something from a shop. Although it is to be hoped that everyone visiting a particular country will do some homework and know a little about the culture they are visiting, it would take years, if not a lifetime, to understand the complexities of other people's cultural behaviour.

True 'cultural enlightenment' may therefore not be obtainable. Perhaps the best that can be achieved is a state of **cultural awareness** (i.e. aware that others may have different beliefs, views and practices from our own) and cultural respect (i.e. respect for those beliefs, even if they are incongruent with our own). This process should, of course, be a two-way street: that is, whereas we may feel we should respect others, it is only fair that they should also respect us.

Phatic communication

Phatic communication is an everyday feature of interaction. First used by the anthropologist Malinowski (1922, 1923) - although he used the phrase 'phatic communion' – the term is used to refer to 'language used in free, aimless, social intercourse' (Malinowski, 1922). Brown and Levinson (1987) observed that, for such talk, 'the subject of talk is not as important as the fact of carrying on a conversation that is amply loaded with . . . markers of emotional agreement'. The *Hutchinson Encyclopaedia* (2000) defines phatic communication as: 'denoting speech as a means of sharing feelings or establishing sociability, rather than for the communication of information and ideas'. We might think of phatic communication as ordinary chat, or 'small talk'.

Examples of phatic communication are scattered throughout most conversations. Most greetings and acknowledgements are phatic. An example of a phatic exchange is as follows:

> **'Hi. How are you getting on?'**
> **'I'm OK thanks. How about you?'**
> **'Yes, fine, thanks.'**
> **'Good. I'm not doing so badly.'**

Note that, in such an exchange, the point is not to establish the health status of the other person but simply to acknowledge their presence and to establish rapport, and that 'we are friends'. In this way, phatic communication can be compared and contrasted with information *requesting and receiving*. In the phatic exchange, the content of the conversation is not important: the point is to establish or re-establish social relationships.

The degree of phatic communication used in any culture probably varies. Sometimes, phatic communication is almost completely devoid of content or formal meaning. Consider, for example, the use of language by young people. It is not uncommon, at present, for younger people to insert the word 'like' into their conversation in a way that has little formal meaning. An example of such use, in a phatic sense, would be the following statement: 'I mean, I was like "wow".'

The statement has little formal content but is used, perhaps, to indicate a certain emotional tone to the listener. Also, a language style that includes the fairly random use of the word 'like' may be adopted by younger people to exclude older people. In this sense, the phatic communication becomes almost a private language, or a means of indicating solidarity between people of the same age. It may also be the language of songs, poetry and 'rapping'.

It seems possible that there is sometimes a 'private language' at work in certain forms of mental illness. Certain types of psychotic state are sometimes characterised by unusual use of language. However, it is perhaps important to distinguish between the 'modern' or 'popular' use of language as used by young people, and the evidence of some cognitive or emotional disturbance displayed by people with problems in living.

Phatic communication is important. Without it, and with only informative communication taking place between two people, conversations would be stark affairs. Consider, for example, the following exchange:

'Do you want to talk?'
'Yes.'
'When?'
'Later.'
'Where?'
'In private.'

This, more normally, is 'padded' with a little phatic communication, perhaps as follows:

> **'Do you want to talk about how you are feeling, at all?'**
> **'Yes, I do, I think . . .'**
> **'When is the best time for you to sit down and talk, do you think?'**
> **'Not at the moment, thanks. I want to be quiet for a bit. Later on this afternoon?'**
> **'Where would you feel most comfortable talking?'**
> **'In private, I think. In your office, perhaps?'**

Much of the above exchange is redundant, as far as understanding and the passing on of information are concerned. However, we are social animals and do not communicate simply to pass on information, but also to develop relationships.

Question for reflection

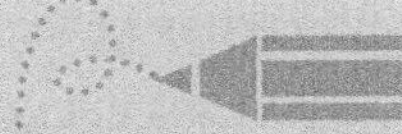

Next time you have a conversation with a friend, colleague or patient, carefully consider how much of the conversation is 'padded out'. What purpose do you think this serves for both parties?

Phatic communication can be helpful in making patients feel comfortable and 'thought about', but it can also be carried on too long. Sometimes, the lack of content of a conversation stops the patient being able to express specifically what they need to say. Nurses might therefore wish to consider pacing their conversations with patients, so that, after a few phatic comments the conversation can be steered towards the essence. For example:

> **'How are you feeling today?'**
> **'Not so bad, thanks.'**
> **'You look better than when I saw you last night.'**
> **'Thanks.'**
> **'Do you still have much pain?'**
> **'I still feel very sore around my stomach . . .'**
> **'Have you had any medication for it recently?'**

'No, I don't like to ask.'
'I will see what you are due or can have.'
'Thank you very much.'

Listening, turn-taking and pacing

In the west, perhaps, particularly in the UK and USA, people tend to pay great attention to listening to one another. Listening is particularly emphasised in counselling, psychotherapy and interpersonal skills training. Being able to listen really well to another person is seen as a great asset. Similarly, and linked to this, is that the same people 'turn take' in conversations. If two people are talking to each other, one will allow the other to finish speaking before offering their own point of view. Further, conversations in the UK and USA are fairly evenly 'paced'. That is to say, they are fairly continuous and are carried on at a regular speed until the conversation ceases. The end of a conversation is clearly marked by both parties saying 'goodbye' or its equivalent.

In the east, none of these rules necessarily applies. In Thailand, conversations between groups of friends are notable by their low volume (people do not shout to be heard) and the fact that, often, many people will be talking at the same time. This may be due to the cultural factors of content and process. In the west it is usually felt important to understand everything that is said: this leads to the listening and turn–taking, described above. There is usually a logical flow to the conversations. This can be described as an emphasis on content. Such discussions often lead to arguments and debates about certain issues. This is not to suggest that they are necessarily hostile, but that, as 'equals', western people often choose to challenge what their friends and colleagues say. In the east, the accent is often on process: it matters, perhaps more than is the case in the west, that everyone is taking part in what is going on. Harmony and agreement are sought where possible, and challenges and debates are not the norm: 'junior' people will necessarily give way to more senior members of the group.

The idea of pacing in conversations tends to reflect similar issues. Conversations and discussions in the west tend towards a linear style of progression: a point is raised, it is discussed, and a means of 'closure' is worked towards. Out of this initial discussion, other issues may be raised and worked through in a similar manner. In the east, however, a conversation or discussion may cover many topics and meander in a way that is not immediately recognisable in the west. This is a roundabout style of communication which can often be noted in Thai speech patterns. The first author has noted that when interviewing Thai students and teachers in research projects, their answers to questions may, indeed, be very roundabout. An answer can start with a 'no' and end with a 'yes'. For example:

> **Researcher: Do you believe in ghosts and spirits?**
> **Respondent: I don't, but older people do and those who live in northern Thailand. It is an old fashioned idea. Sometimes I believe it a little, and I respect ghosts and they scare me. Yes, I do believe in them.**

Practice-based Case Study

Acute surgical pain in an elderly patient from South-east Asia

I work as a staff nurse on a general surgical ward in a district general hospital in south Wales, UK. For almost a year I have worked with a qualified nursing colleague who was recruited by the hospital directly from South-east Asia. Several months ago his parents came to stay with him and his wife for 2 weeks, before paying a visit to his other brother (also a registered nurse) in the USA. However, a few days before they were due to leave the UK, his mother developed severe abdominal pain and was admitted to our ward with appendicitis. She was taken to theatre that evening for an appendectomy, and returned to the ward in the early hours of the morning.

My colleague Jeff* (*a pseudonym) was not allowed to work on the ward while his mother was an in-patient. The first morning, I cared for Jeff's mother. While walking around the ward to assess the patients under my care, I spoke with her and asked her if she had any pain. She responded, 'No, I am fine', to which I replied, 'Well if you do have any pain, please let me know and I can give you some painkillers, if you think you need them'. I then left her and spent

some time with the other patients, but when I later left the bed area to answer the phone, I saw her holding her abdomen and grimacing.

I made my way to her bed and asked her how she was feeling. She again replied 'Fine', although her body language suggested otherwise. I therefore commented that I thought she looked uncomfortable and asked her if she was now experiencing any pain. However, she again replied, 'No, I'm fine', but because of her behaviour I was not convinced and felt that she probably was experiencing some discomfort. I then looked at her drug chart and discovered that she had not had any analgesia for over 6 hours, but obviously I did not want to keep asking her the same question over and over again.

I therefore took a different approach and sat at the side of her bed and started to talk about how she felt in general. We quickly struck up a conversation about how she was feeling, and soon established a rapport. At this point, I gently asked her if she was uncomfortable, to which she finally admitted that she was 'quite uncomfortable'. When I asked her why she had not told me sooner, she replied that she did not want to bother me. I immediately arranged some analgesia for her and emphasised the importance of her telling me if she was experiencing any discomfort in the future.

I didn't think any more about the incident until Jeff arrived on the ward later in the day with his wife and father to visit his mother. We spoke together and I explained how his mother was doing, and I briefly mentioned the incident to him. I felt that, as with many patients, especially the elderly, it was probably due to the fact that she just didn't want to 'trouble me'. However, Jeff explained to me that this 'roundabout' form of communication (particularly the apparent switching from no to yes (or vice versa) and back again) is found in many cultures, especially those in South-east Asia, but is almost never seen in northern Europe, the USA or the UK.

On reflection, I suppose that this particular incident is, perhaps, an important issue in cross-cultural nursing. However, I was unaware of this type of behaviour and probably would never have found out about it, unless I'd experienced it first hand. What it did make me realise, though, was the importance of using a range of communication skills, especially when caring for those from a different culture. It really made me think about how, as nurses, we should communicate with patients in order to acquire important information from them. I am now aware that good communication is not just about talking, or even listening: it's also about observing and assessing the situation, so that you use the most appropriate approach and skills (verbal and non-verbal) in that situation.

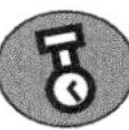

Direct and indirect communication

Cultures vary in the degree to which their members communicate directly or indirectly. In the USA and the UK it is fairly common for people to express their views and preferences quite directly (as in, 'Yes, I like that', or 'No, I don't like that'). In many cultures, however, communication is much less direct (for example in South-east Asia) and opinions are rarely expressed so as to avoid offending the other person.

Speaking indirectly and not expressing strong opinions is a way of increasing social cohesion. What is more important is what the group thinks, rather than what 'I' think. Another example of this everyday directness and indirectness can be observed by comparing and contrasting UK and Thai people looking around the shops. The UK person will tend to turn to his or her companion and say about something in a shop window: 'That is beautiful', or 'That is so ugly'. A Thai person, however, is more likely simply to point to something in a shop window and make no comment. Usually, interestingly, their 'opinion' is often conveyed, perhaps by a smile or by a smirk, but an outright comment on what is being looked at is rarer.

Related to this is the amount that is spoken. North American and British people tend to feel a need to talk, and will often extract every last detail out of a description or a discussion. South-east Asian people, however, will often be much quieter and feel the need to talk only when there is 'something to say'. Part of this, too, may relate to Buddhist tradition, in which to be quiet and thoughtful of others are important values.

Compliments

Cultures vary in the ways in which they treat or give compliments. In UK culture it is common to belittle a compliment once it is given. It is not unusual for the hearer to dismiss the compliment with a phrase such as 'not really', whereas in other cultures it is not uncommon for compliments to be returned. Valdes (1986) gives the following example of a conversation between two Iranian friends:

> **'Your shoes are nice'.**
> **'It is your eyes which can see them that are nice.'**

As a rule, Thai people seem to enjoy paying each other, and other people, compliments.

Answering questions

In a UK or North American context, people expect others to answer questions clearly and unambiguously. In some cultures, however, it is considered rude to say 'no' as an answer to a question. The Japanese 'no', for example, if given at all, will be given with a sigh, indicating the speaker's reluctance to use it. The Chinese 'no' is more likely to be worded as 'That may be difficult', to avoid the problem (Varner and Beamer, 1995).

Similarly, in some cultures giving very direct answers to questions, if those questions are posed by persons of senior status, is frowned upon. Again, 'no' answers are often given only very reluctantly. Further, students may worry about offering a 'challenging' response to a teacher's question in class. Someone from a South-east Asian background is likely to be loath to force a teacher to question his own statements, as to do so would mean loss of face on the part of both the student and the teacher. This goes some way to meet the criticism, often heard in UK nursing colleges, that 'overseas students won't criticise or debate issues in class'.

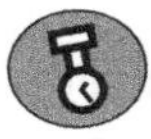

Similarities in communication

Despite cultural differences, there are some behaviours and ways of communicating that seem to be universal. Almost all cultures appreciate politeness and respect between communicators (Brown and Levinson, 1987).

Most languages have an equivalent of 'hello' as a form of greeting, and have rules about the freedom with which people can use forms of other people's names. Using given names is usually the prerogative of friends and seniors (however, in Thailand, for example, given names are used routinely but may be prefaced by a title: 'Mr David', or 'Professor Sarah').

In most cultural groups it is appreciated if the visitor or foreigner attempts to use the local language. British and North American people have probably become lazy about learning other languages because of the seeming universality of the use of English. If the visitor moves out of large cities and into rural environments, however, it quickly becomes clear that English is not so 'universally' spoken.

The process of learning cultural differences – in both communication and more generally – is not always without pain and a certain sense of loss. The 'enculturation process' (a process of cultural adaptation) can also involve a loss of one's own sense of culture, as Hoffman (1989) so graphically illustrates in this description by a Polish student living in England:

> ***My mother says I'm becoming English. This hurts me, because I know she means I'm becoming cold. I'm no colder than I've ever been, but I'm learning to be less demonstrative. I learn this from a teacher who, after contemplating the gesticulations with which I help myself describe the digestive system of a frog, tells me to 'sit on my hands and then try talking'. I learn my new reserve from people who take a step back when we talk because I'm standing too close, crowding them. Cultural distances are different. I learn in a sociology class, but I know it already . . .*** *(Hoffman, 1989)*

Although the examples in this book, which have been used to highlight some of the cultural differences in communication, have often been drawn from what traditionally have been called 'east' and 'west', it is not particularly helpful or accurate to think in these terms, especially as most societies, including the UK, are now multicultural. Therefore, most nurses are likely to come into contact with patients from other societies or cultures, who may, on occasion or in certain circumstances, communicate differently.

Although differences between cultures are often most noticeable between those physically distanced from each other, this need not be the case: the French, for example, usually shake hands on meeting friends; British people tend not to do so with the same frequency.

Proximity

Proximity refers to the distance we maintain when we stand or sit in relation to each other when we talk. There are considerable cultural variations in this. For example, people in Latin countries, such as Spain and Italy, tend to stand closer together than do people from the UK. It is even possible to experiment with proximity. Next time you are talking to a friend, take half a step towards them. You will probably find that your friend takes a small step backwards, in order to find their 'comfort zone'. It is possible to move people considerable distances by gradually moving towards them as you converse.

Those in dominant positions may overestimate the degree to which they can stand close to a person in a more subservient position. Thus 'the boss' may stand closer to an employee than is comfortable for the latter. Similarly, nurses (who, by the nature of their jobs, are in a dominant position) may stand too close to patients. For the patient who is in bed, too, the nurse may get too close. It is important to consider proximity, to be aware of it, and to allow the other person to find their own comfort zone when you are chatting. A useful device for nurses who meet patients in outpatients or clinics is to invite them to 'pull your chair over', which will allow them to set a comfortable distance. Note that even this suggestion has cultural implications. In Thailand, for example, sliding a chair across the ground is considered rude.

Touch

Cultures vary in the degree to which they use touch as a form of communication. Many Latin countries are 'high touch' countries, where it is normal to be able to touch the other person during a conversation, particularly when reassuring someone. In most western countries, an initial, albeit formal, greeting is the handshake. In Islamic countries, the opposite of these is true: informal touch is rare and touch between the sexes is usually forbidden. It is not acceptable, in most Islamic countries, for example, for a man to shake hands with women. However, this rule is not universal. In the Islamic sultanate of Brunei, it is reasonably common for men to be able to shake hands with women. In Thailand, the handshake is common, but not as common between Thais as the *wai*: a prayer-like gesture of the hands. The *wai* is offered by the junior person to the more senior, and it is not usual to wai people for services rendered. For example, it would be considered odd to return a waiter's *wai* as he thanks you for eating at his restaurant.

The *wai* has many other meanings beyond that of a greeting, and is used in countries other than Thailand. It can also be used to indicate that 'I am sorry'. It is not uncommon to see a Thai driver apologising to another with a *wai* when the first mentioned has broken one of the rules of the road. This is interesting, given that many Thai drivers break most of the rules of the road.

In some countries the head is considered a sacred part of the body and the feet are considered dirty. It is therefore considered a great rudeness to touch the head of another, or to point with the feet or touch someone else with the feet. Again, these rules apply in Thailand. However, those in certain professions, such as nursing, are (very practically) allowed to break these taboos and can touch the head or the feet without apology. Other health-care professionals, such as doctors and masseurs, are also freed from this rule.

Eye contact

The degree to which eye contact is maintained or initiated varies from country to country and from culture to culture. In the west, and, perhaps particularly in the USA, it is not uncommon for two people talking to one another to maintain fairly constant eye contact. However, in the east, the more senior person in a pair is allowed to make eye contact with the more junior, but the more junior will often frequently look down as a mark of respect. In the east, it is usually rare to make continuous eye contact.

In most parts of the world, eye contact is made at the beginning of an utterance, and as the person continues to say what he or she is saying, they look away. However, for a reason I have never been able to identify, in the Caribbean this rule is reversed. The person looks away as he or she starts an utterance and looks towards the person as he or she continues the conversation.

Volume and gesture

People in different countries vary in the volume at which they pitch their speech. Perhaps the 'loudest' people in the world are those from Latin countries and those from the USA. British people can talk loudly but often adopt moderate volume levels. Many people in South-east Asia talk very quietly, and this can be a problem for nurses working with or caring for people from this part of the world. As well as trying to understand English spoken with a broad accent, the UK nurse may have problems hearing what is being said. Again, hierarchy comes into play here. A junior person from South-east Asia will often talk more quietly than a more senior person, out of due respect.

Use of gesture as a means of communicating varies considerably from culture to culture. Compare, for example, Italian and Thai use of hand and arm gestures. Italians often use hand gestures to a very large degree while conversing, and, because of the volume of their conversation, it is possible to think that they are arguing. Conversely, when Thais talk they use very little hand movement: 'talking' is conversation, as it were. Similarly, in formal settings in the UK, few hand movements are made. Until recently, television newsreaders and reporters used very little hand movement.

Conclusion

This chapter has explored the concept of communication, including the intricacies and subtle nuances associated with communication in a cultural context and the potential impact these issues can have on nursing practice.

Suggested reading

Burnard P (2002). *Learning Human Skills: an Experiential and Reflective Guide for Nurses and Health Care Professionals*, 4th edn. Oxford: Butterworth-Heinemann.

Clarke L (2001). *Contemporary Nursing: Culture, Education and Practice*. London: APS.

Dutta M (2007). *Communicating Health: a Culture–centred Approach*. London: Polity Press.

Leininger M (2001). *Culture, Care Diversity and Universality: a Theory of Nursing*. New York: Jones and Bartlett.

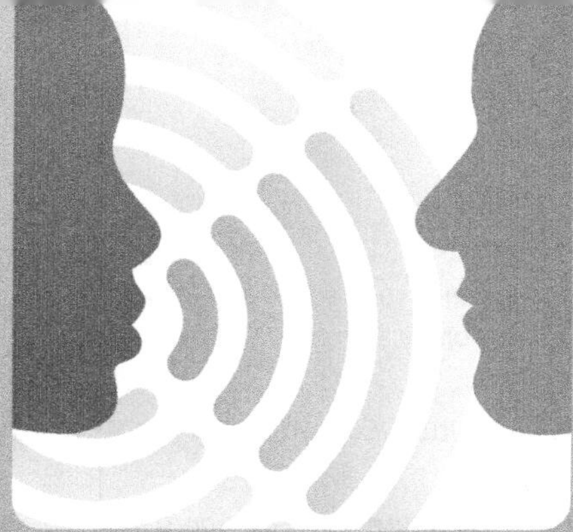

Chapter 3

Communication skills

Learning outcomes

At the end of this chapter, you should be able to:

- ✔ identify a range of communication skills
- ✔ discuss listening in the role of communication
- ✔ identify cultural issues in the communication process

Introduction

This chapter explores communication skills commonly used by nurses in everyday practice, and focuses specifically on listening and verbal communication skills.

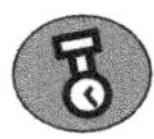

Communication skills in nursing

Listening

To listen to another person is the most human of actions. In nursing it is the crucial skill. Listening refers to the process of *hearing* what the client is saying. Hearing encompasses not only the words that are being used, but also the non-verbal aspects of the encounter. Thus attending refers to a person's skill in paying attention to the other person and keeping their attention 'focused out' and completely on that person.

So why listen? Hargie, Saunders and Dickson (1994) list the general functions of listening as follows:

1. To focus specifically upon the messages being communicated by the other person
2. To obtain a full, accurate understanding of the other person's communication
3. To convey interest, concern and attention
4. To encourage full, open and honest expression
5. To develop an 'other-centred' approach during an interaction.

Listening: a skill or a quality?

In a study of UK nursing students, Burnard (1998) surveyed some of them about their perception of the qualities of a nurse acting as a counsellor. The term 'counsellor', in this case, was defined as 'the sort that a person might go to see to talk about personal or emotional problems'. This was to differentiate between a counsellor as helper and confidante and other sorts of counsellors, such as coaches, information givers, trainers and supervisors.

Two groups of pre-registration nurses, on a range of courses in a school of nursing in Cardiff, were surveyed (a total of 200 students). Students could choose whether or not they completed the form, which asked them to list the qualities that they associated with effective counselling communication. They were asked only to identify qualities and not skills.

One hundred and sixty-two usable survey papers were returned, a response rate of 81%.

Among the most frequently identified qualities were those broadly in line with previous research and the literature: being non-judgemental, being empathic, and being understanding. However, other qualities, such as being approachable, sympathetic and caring, rated highly too. Often, **empathy** is identified in the literature as an important personal quality, whereas sympathy is not. However, these items represent abstractions and, as such, may be difficult to define clearly. Safety and ethical qualities also appeared to be important (such as being confidential, trustworthy and honest). It should be noted, too, that some respondents addressed the issue in terms of 'negatives' (e.g. counsellors should be non-threatening, non-patronising, or not forceful). The surprise 'quality', perhaps, was *good listener:* 73% of the sample identified this as a personal quality. As we shall see, in the discussion below this runs counter to much of the literature, which defines listening as a skill rather than as a quality. Table 3.1 identifies the range of findings down to qualities identified by at least five respondents.

Discussion

The findings highlight an interesting ambiguity. Although the literature on counselling often identifies listening as a skill (see, for example, Davis and Fallowfield, 1991, Morrison and Burnard, 1991), many of the respondents in this study identified it as a *personal* quality. This is all the more clearly underlined by the fact that, at the top of the response sheet, was the indication that the researcher was interested only in personal *qualities* and not in skills, as discussed above. It is made more interesting by the fact that no other skills were identified in this way. If the respondents were generally mistaking or confusing qualities for skills, it would be likely that they would also identify other skills in this way.

Effective listening behaviours

Egan (1982) offers a useful acronym for remembering the important aspects of non-verbal activity during the listening process. He argues that, in western countries, these behaviours are usually associated with effective listening.

Table 3.1 Qualities of nurse-counsellors as identified by students (n = 162)

Quality	n	%
Good listener	119	73
Non-judgemental	93	57
Empathic	56	35
Understanding	56	35
Approachable	43	27
Sympathetic	32	20
Caring	31	19
Friendly	31	19
Patient	28	17
Confidential	27	17
Supportive	22	14
Knowledgeable	19	12
Honest	18	11
Trustworthy	16	10
Experienced	12	7
Kind	12	7
Warm	12	7
Calm	11	7
Helpful	9	6
Respectful	8	5
Sense of humour	8	5
Advice giving	7	4
Considerate	7	4
Genuine	7	4
Open	7	4
Open-minded	7	4
Professional	7	4
Non-patronising	6	4
Objective	6	4
Reassuring	6	4
Trusting	6	4
Broad-minded	5	3
Comforting	5	3
Communicative	5	3
Relaxed	5	3

Case Study

Culture and nursing: a Bruneian nurse's perceptions

I live in a culture-sensitive society. Culture and religion play an important part and most of the time influence my daily life, including my work as a nurse. It is difficult not to mention religion when writing about culture. This is because some religious practices become part of a culture. One example is visiting a sick person in hospital. Every nursing textbook says that hospital wards should be as quiet as possible. This is necessary for recovery, even though this means separation from family and friends. In my religion [Islam], and because of being part of a culture, the sick person should be supported by the presence of their family and is never left alone, or allowed to die without members of the family present. Therefore, as a nurse, it is quite difficult for me when the whole family of the patient wishes to be involved in the care of their loved one. When I say the whole family, I mean from the grandparents to the grandchildren. It is very common to see wards in Brunei hospitals packed with family members visiting their loved ones.

Another traditional example of our belief and culture is that we should do good things with the right hand. For example, if I want to give an injection to the patient, I am expected to do it with the right hand. This is not an issue for right-handed nurses, but for the left-handed like me can be a problem. Sometimes I have to ask permission from the patient to use the left hand. Fortunately, I have never come across a patient who refused to be injected by a left-handed nurse.

The nursing textbooks that I read are published in Europe, such as the United Kingdom, and the USA. Therefore, my nursing education and knowledge are very much based on western ideas. In the textbooks it says that we should have good eye contact while communicating with the patient. I am not arguing with this because it is true. However, in my culture we need to control our eye contact while talking to other people, especially with the opposite sex and the elderly. Direct eye contact can sometimes be interpreted as rude.

One very interesting area that I should not forget to mention is sexuality. When I was a student, I learned about Nancy Roper's Activities of Daily Living model. We are expected to use this model in clinical practice. One of the activities in that model is expressing sexuality. Theoretically, it is not difficult for me if my teacher asks me to write about how to assess the needs of patients regarding expressing sexuality. However, to put it into practice is very, very difficult, because sexuality is such a sensitive issue in our culture. Therefore, this activity is almost never assessed in our patients, and rarely discussed.

I think nurses should have an open mind and be fully aware of their own cultural beliefs. Then they will be able and willing to respect the individual patient, regardless of their cultural practices and beliefs.

Roper N **et al.** (1996). *The Elements of Nursing. A Model for Nursing Based on a Model of Living*, 4th edn. New York: Churchill Livingstone.

The **listening behaviours** that Egan identifies are:

- **S - Sit squarely in relation to the other person**
- **O - Maintain an 'open' position and do not cross arms or legs**
- **L - Lean slightly towards the other person**
- **E - Maintain reasonable and comfortable eye contact**
- **R - Relax.**

Egan's guidelines on how to sit when listening may be useful as a baseline for thinking about listening to another person. It also has applications in the teaching of more effective communication skills. On the other hand, we might also notice some (North American) culture bias in these guidelines. The amount of eye contact that is made in two-way conversations varies considerably between cultures. Not all students or junior nurses from different cultures will, for example, be happy with constantly maintained eye contact, and may prefer rather more occasional eye contact. Nor will they automatically maintain eye contact themselves in the presence of someone they perceive as being senior to them.

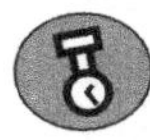 Verbal communication skills

A format for understanding the range of communication skills was devised by Heron (1989) and is called **Six Category Intervention Analysis**. This was offered as a conceptual model for understanding interpersonal relationships, and as an assessment tool for identifying a range of possible interactions between two people. The six categories are: prescriptive (offering advice); informative (offering information); confronting (challenging); cathartic (enabling the expression of pent-up emotions); catalytic ('drawing out'); and supportive (confirming or encouraging). The word 'intervention' is used to describe any statement that the practitioner may use. The word 'category' is used to denote a range of related interventions.

Heron (1989) calls the first three categories (prescriptive, informative and confronting) 'authoritative', and suggests that by using them the *practitioner* retains control over the relationship. He calls the second three categories (cathartic, catalytic and supportive) 'facilitative', and suggests that these enable the *client* to retain control over the relationship. In other words, the first three are 'practitioner-centred' and the second three are 'client-centred'. Another way of describing the difference between these sets of categories is that the first three are 'You tell me' interventions and the second three are 'I tell you' interventions.

What, then, is the value of such an analysis of communication skills? First, it identifies the range of possible interventions available to the nurse. Very often, in day-to-day interactions with others, we stick to repetitive forms of conversation and response simply because we are not aware that other options are available. This analysis identifies an exhaustive range of types of human intervention. Second, by identifying the sorts of interventions we can use, we can act more precisely and with a greater sense of intention. The nurse-patient relationship thus becomes more particular and less haphazard: we know *what* we are saying and also *how* we are saying it. We have greater interpersonal choice.

Questions for reflection

Consider the very first time a patient asked you about their condition, prognosis and associated treatment. How did you deal with this encounter? In particular, how did you communicate with the patient (verbally and non-verbally)? Also, how does this incident compare to how you would now handle such a situation?

Third, the analysis offers an instrument for training. Once the categories have been identified, they can be used for students and others to identify their weaknesses and strengths across the interpersonal spectrum. In this way, nurses can develop a wide and comprehensive range of interpersonal skills (Burnard, 2002).

UK nurses' perceptions of their interpersonal skills

In two studies (Burnard and Morrison, 1988, Morrison and Burnard, 1991), UK student nurses and trained nursing staff were asked to rate their communication skills in terms of the Six Category Intervention Analysis. In the first study, using an accidental sample of 92 trained nurses, the nurses were asked to rank order the six categories according to how skilful they thought they were in using them. Generally speaking, the nurses perceived themselves to be more skilled in using the authoritative categories and less skilled in using the facilitative categories. Having said that, most of the nurses perceived themselves as being particularly weak in using cathartic and catalytic interventions. Overall, they perceived themselves as being best at being supportive.

There were marked similarities in the findings of the second study, in which 84 student nurses were invited to rank order the six categories in terms of their perceived strengths and weaknesses in using them. Again, we found an overall picture of greater perceived skill in using authoritative interventions rather than facilitative ones. Students also thought that they were generally most effective in using supportive interventions and not so good at using cathartic and confronting interventions. In general, the results of both studies support Heron's (1989) assertion that a wide range of practitioners in our society show a much greater deficit in the skilful use of facilitative interventions than they do in the skilful use of authoritative ones.

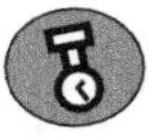

Six Category Intervention Analysis: a cultural perspective

Prescriptive

It should be noted that in many cultures, patients expect health-care professionals (particularly doctors) to be prescriptive. In these cultures the doctor is the 'expert' and is highly respected. It would not be normal or appropriate to challenge the doctor's suggestions, and those suggestions are usually closely followed by patients.

Similarly, in nursing education the teacher is someone who is listened to and their suggestions are acted upon. Again, the teacher is the expert, and it is not for the student to challenge what they say.

Informative

Again, in a number of cultures, information given by health-care professionals is expected to be both wise and accurate. It is not to be challenged (for example, see the Practice-based Case Study below). In the west, patients (and students) have become familiar with patient-centred and student-centred approaches to health and education. This is certainly not the case in large parts of the world. Similarly, western students are likely to have been encouraged to think critically. Nursing students and practitioners coming from Asia are less likely to engage in this style of education. For them, it is more likely that the nurse educator is the one who has the 'right answers', and similarly it is the health-care professional who has the information they need.

Doctor–patient communication in Africa

In the late 1990s I left the UK to work on a 1-year project for the United Nations Children's Fund (UNICEF) in Eastern and Southern Africa. I was based primarily in Kenya, promoting children's health in local health centres. The health professionals that I worked with came from all over the world, including France, the UK, North America and Africa.

One day I was working in a clinic in Nairobi with a young physician called Steve* (*a pseudonym), who was born, educated and trained in Africa. He was very pleasant, but his approach to dealing with patients was what I, as a British nurse, considered to be 'old school', i.e. he talked, they listened, and I then ensured that they understood what had been said. On this particular day a young mother came to clinic with her son for a routine immunisation programme. She arrived in clinic while Steve was still talking to another doctor in the centre, so we quickly struck up a conversation in his absence. It transpired that she was a teacher and had been trained and educated in the UK, where she had also worked for some time, before returning to Kenya because of her husband's job. She appeared to be far more educated and affluent than many of the families who would normally attend this health centre.

Steve then came back into the room, where he introduced himself to the mother and child. He quickly asked some routine health questions and then recommended to the mother an immunisation programme for her child. He briefly provided some supporting verbal information, and then stood to go and see another mother and child in the adjacent area. However, before he could leave, the woman asked him some specific questions about possible side effects and contraindications of the immunisation programme. Steve was very taken aback and looked clearly flustered. Although he did answer her questions, his body language, response and tone of voice clearly indicated his annoyance. I also spoke with the woman, before administering the first prescribed immunisation medication. When we were alone, she laughed to me about this incident and explained that 'the doctors over here are not used to people, especially women, asking them questions'.

Later Steve asked me, 'Why do these people ask the doctor so many questions, instead of just listening?' I explained to him that she had lived and been educated in the UK, and that in the west, questioning health professionals is normal and does not necessarily demonstrate distrust or disrespect, but is essential to understanding treatment and forms an important aspect of the informed consent process. He simply nodded, shrugged and walked off.

Although I have no wish to be negative, I am not really sure whether Steve really understood what I had told him. However, the lesson for me, as a nurse, from this incident was that communication needs, practices and expectations vary from person to person, regardless of culture. Therefore, the challenge for nurses and other health professionals, particularly when working with those from other cultures, is to try and recognise what these needs are and, if possible, to communicate in the most effective way.

Confronting

In many cultures, confrontation works 'down the hierarchy'. A senior student nurse can confront a junior student nurse; a doctor can confront a nurse. For many people in the world, it is simply not acceptable to think of confronting senior people.

Catalytic

Not everyone in the world sees sharing their problems as the way to deal with them. In the west, it is common for a friend – and particularly for a counsellor – to 'draw out' a person with problems in order for that person to express themselves more clearly. This is seen as a necessary step towards problem solving and is summed up by the expression: 'a problem shared is a problem halved'. Again, however, this is not a universal point of view. In Thailand, for example, it is not considered polite to share your problems with others. This is part of the quality known as *kreng jai* – of putting other peoples' feelings before your own. A Thai person, then, will embarrass a friend if they encourage them to share their problems, but is more likely to jolly them along to distract them. Disclosing one's problems is not the norm in Thailand.

Cathartic

Again, in the west, and perhaps particularly in the United States, it is felt important for people to express their feelings: 'Better out than in' is a saying about feelings that many people would concur with. However, in the east it is often considered quite inappropriate to show feelings openly, even among family and friends. Research into how student nurses in Brunei handled stress and emotional distress found that many would find other ways of dealing with emotional pain, but they would not willingly express their feelings to others (see more about this later in the book). Similarly, in Thailand it is considered that a person who openly expresses emotion is going against the concept of *kreng jai* (the Thai idea that we should put others before ourselves).

A further issue in Thai culture is that expressing anger is particularly looked down upon. The expression of anger is considered animal behaviour, and in Buddhist cosmology constantly demonstrating animal behaviour in a human context may mean that a person will return as an animal in a future life. Either way, losing your temper or showing aggressive feelings is a certain way of alienating your friends and sometimes your family. If you show aggression it will mean that you have 'lost the argument'.

Supportive

Most cultures encourage people to support each other, although the amount of support offered may depend on your position in society. In nursing education in Thailand, and unlike the situation in the UK, nurse teachers are ***in loco parentis***, or acting as parents to their students. It is expected that nurse teachers in Thailand will be extremely supportive and encouraging of their students, and often appear to act (to the western viewer) in a 'parental' way. In the UK and in the USA, students are generally thought to be adults and are usually treated as such. They are also expected to be independent learners and may not be offered the detailed support offered to Thai students.

Conclusion

This chapter has explored communication skills used in nursing. The next chapter is based on an empirical study into culture and communication in Thai nursing.

Suggested reading

Burnard P (2005). *Counselling Skills for Health Professionals*, 4th edn. Gloucester: Nelson Thornes.

Ellis R, Gates B and Kenworthy N (2003). *Interpersonal Communication in Nursing*, 2nd edn. Edinburgh: Churchill Livingstone.

McCabe C and Timmins F (2006). *Communication Skills for Nursing Practice*. Basingstoke: Palgrave.

Riley J B (2007). *Communication in Nursing*. London: Mosby.

Sully P and Dallas J (2005). *Essential Communication Skills for Nursing Practice*. London: Mosby.

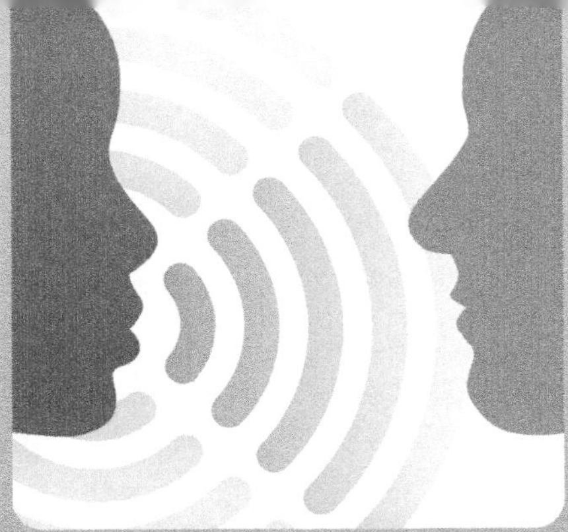

Chapter 4

Culture and communication in Thai nursing: an example of a different culture

Learning outcomes

At the end of this chapter, you should be able to:

- ✔ compare and contrast your own views about communication and nursing with Thai communication and culture
- ✔ think about cultural differences in nursing care
- ✔ consider whether or not you have ethnocentric views about nursing and communication.

Introduction

This chapter offers some key findings of an ethnographic study into culture and communication in Thai nursing (Burnard and Naiyapatana, 2004). The study took place in Thailand, and a small number of nurses, nurse educators, lay people and a Buddhist monk were interviewed. The study also included participant observation (including general observations of everyday life in Thailand), and the findings reported here are from both the interviews and observations.

The purpose of this chapter is to provide a more detailed insight into aspects of nursing and communication in another country. It is hoped that by providing an ethnographic case study, it will allow the reader to compare and contrast social and cultural similarities and differences (particularly in relation to nursing, health and illness) in Thailand and their own country. It should be pointed out that this chapter is by no means exhaustive, and although many of the issues discussed are relatively common in Thai society, we do not suggest that the findings can or should be generalised.

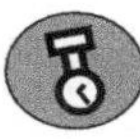

Background to the study

The study was conducted by the first author (PB), in collaboration with a Thai nursing colleague, Dr Wassana Naiyapatana. The aim was to explore the ways in which Thai cultural issues influence interpersonal communication patterns in Thai nursing and nursing education. However, although the focus of the study was on communication in Thai nursing, many of the fundamental issues that subsequently emerged relate directly to Thai culture as a whole, for example Buddhism, family friends, and social and cultural issues associated with Thai life in general. Many of the issues, therefore, are inextricably intertwined and reflect on Thai culture as a whole, not just nursing.

There were a number of reasons for undertaking this study. First, it provided some insight into the styles of nursing used in other parts of the world. Second, partly due to the world shortage of nurses, and nurses' increasing ability to work in other countries, it helped improve understanding of different nursing contexts. Nursing involves communication more than almost any other element of behaviour and action. For those who choose to work in Thailand, or perhaps for those nurses who work with Thai nurses elsewhere in the world, it is helpful to understand aspects of the culture. Third, student nurses often visit other countries as part of their initial degree programmes, and it can help them significantly if they have an understanding of the culture in which they may choose to work. Finally, in understanding about communication in different cultures, we often learn more about ourselves and our own ways of communicating with staff and patients.

Twelve participants (nurse educators and clinical nurses) were recruited from a Thai college of nursing. Data were collected primarily through semistructured interviews. Interviews were conducted in English and lasted for approximately 40–60 minutes. Field notes were also compiled. Data were analysed using a form of thematic content analysis (Burnard, 1991) using the data analysis software Atlas ti. This chapter is therefore organised mainly under the headings of relevant key themes.

Permission to interview the respondents from the college of nursing was granted at a local level in Thailand. Participants were assured of anonymity and confidentiality, and were informed about the purpose and nature of the study. They were also informed that they could withdraw from the interview or the study at any time.

Question for reflection

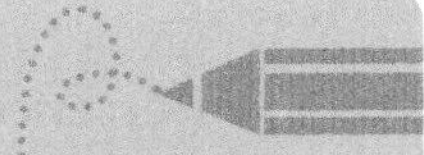

As you read these findings, identify the ways in which nursing in Thailand seems to be similar to and different from nursing in your own country. How do you feel about these similarities and differences?

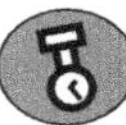

Communication: the interviews

A point needs to be made about the 'oddness' of the relationships between interviewers and those interviewed, in a Thai context. It is not usual for Thai people to talk openly or publicly about their thoughts and feelings. Thai people keep their thoughts to themselves and tend not to bother other people with them. In the interview, however, the informer is being asked to set aside this cultural norm and to 'say anything' (Kvale, 1996). Various problems arise here. First, at least one of the interviewers was an 'outsider' – a foreigner, and someone who did not work in the organisation. Furthermore, as a professor, he may have been ascribed fairly high status, and this may have made it more difficult for others to talk to him, especially 'openly'.

Sometimes, attempts were made to convey a 'good' picture of the subject matter under consideration. When asked about nurses and their communication styles with patients, for example, it was common to get the response: 'They are all treated equally'. However, as the conversation developed, this view would sometimes be moderated by the informant, often along very tentative lines ('Well, perhaps there are times when *some* patients are treated better than others . . .'). No one should doubt that interviews, like all other forms of communication, are to a greater or lesser degree 'stage managed' by those who take part in them. Even the data arising out of interviews are 'confidential' in nature: the uttering of the material that will become data still has to be done by a person who is at the same time presenting a picture of themselves to the interviewer (Wengraf, 2001). Also, the perceived status of the interviewers (a university professor and a senior nursing instructor) may have meant that those being interviewed felt, initially at least, a little intimidated.

There were occasions when the interviewers doubted whether they had got beyond the superficial, 'organisation-positive' view. Some informants were keen to present themselves as 'modern' Thais, to a degree that sometimes sounded exaggerated. Others were keen to stress how 'good' nurses were, and their accounts seemed uncritical. We can probably assume that there are always going to be good and bad nurses in Thailand, as in the rest of the world. Reluctance to criticise, to a 'stranger', may well have contributed to this presentation.

The point, of course, is that these issues regarding interviewing in Thailand are another aspect of 'culture and communication' – the focal point of this study and this book.

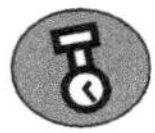

Communicating Thainess

Thai people

The key to understanding something of Thailand is to understand Thai people. In this study, informants were easily able to articulate what it meant to be Thai. Clusters of qualities were often offered together. For example, common characteristics of Thai people were described as friendly, sincere, proud, polite, patient and willing to help. Being Thai was also seen as important, as was **religion** (Buddhism) and the general way of life:

Thais, living in Thailand, always think of themselves as being Thai Buddhist. The monarchy and the king are important. Families are different to, say, Japanese and other SE Asian cultures - Thais are slower than those other cultures. The Japanese and things are more energetic. We are less active and more easy going.

The issue of Thai children looking after their parents was noted by many informants, often in the context of pointing out that western people did not do this. Respecting and caring for the elderly was fundamental.

Despite the fact that some commentators have argued that there are four distinct cultures in Thailand, based on regions, this was denied by one informant:

Thai people are conservative. They change slowly. Although there are regional variations of Thailand, there is not much difference, culturally. All share similar culture.

The issues of personal freedom and social responsibility were often discussed. The idea that the name Thailand meant 'Land of Freedom' was also noted, along with issues regarding the socialisation of children. Comparisons were also made with western cultures, and the economic difficulties of being Thai were noted:

Freedom is the root of the word Thai. Thai means freedom or independence. We have never been colonised. The west

has influenced us a lot, but it causes conflict. What do we choose? We sometimes see ourselves as inferior to western people. They are superior. We have less capacity to think on our own, to improve ourselves. It is to do with economics. We don't have money. We have to depend on the west, and that makes us feel less confident. Conservative does not mean slow to change. Most Thai people would like to keep Thai culture with technology and modern things, alongside families and the social network.

However, key aspects of Thai society, particularly social networks, which were always traditionally strong, were now perceived to be changing. Families tend to take care of each other, and the young, especially, often look after their parents. However, partly due to the economic problems in Thailand, many people have had to move further afield to find work, often breaking up close family networks. Thus was noted the changing nature of Thai culture, the development, perhaps, of nuclear families at the expense of extended ones, and the suggested fear that children might not continue to look after their parents.

Thai people are changing quickly now. They are trying to be western. They want to be free and independent. They think that western young people have more freedom to do what they like.

Not expressing strong feelings is a Thai characteristic, arising perhaps out of Buddhist beliefs and teachings. It was noted here as an important element of being Thai.

Thai people think first before they speak. Do not express emotions. Do not say "I love you". Thais in classroom stay quiet and think about question. US people say whatever they think and do not think about others. Thais are sensitive to others.

In not expressing personal feelings for others and not saying 'I love you', Thai people demonstrate the Buddhist quality of 'non-attachment'. As we have seen, non-attachment is not just for objects and things, but for people too. Acceptance and non-attachment also affected people's reaction to pain.

Control feelings. Older people keep feelings inside. Older patients have more experience and their experience might help communication. Younger people might need more information. Coping with pain . . . Thai people cope with pain easily because of their need not to worry other people.

The 'present-centred' nature of some Thai people was also reflected, as was another form of acceptance of things as they are. Not 'standing out' from others was important.

We do not think about the future. Whatever will be will be, and we can accept it. We have to plan for our lives, but not too high and not too much.

Thais and foreigners

When comparisons were made with 'foreigners' (i.e. those not from Thailand) and with the west, the 'west' was almost always the United States of America. Many of the clinical nurses and nurse educators had completed higher degrees, including doctorates, in the USA. Various characteristics and behaviours of America and North Americans were noted. For example, America was perceived to be more organised, and the people were often seen as being good, systematic, expressive of their feelings (unlike Thais, who often do not express their feelings) and punctual (a reference to the distinction that can be made between 'Thai time' and 'western time', where 'western time' means being punctual). However, issues were noted about racial and religious intolerance in the USA, and the fact that, whereas Thais have a close, extended family, western families are very often independent and not so close.

Differences between Thai and western people are in the way they act, think and speak. North Americans, for example, are more creative and systematic. They have a different language. Thais speak more quietly. It has a background in Buddhism. Non-Thai people do not worry about seniority in the way that Thai people do.

Comparisons, though, were sometimes linked to fears of the Thai culture changing, perhaps as the result of western influences. In the following quote, the informant notes the changes in Thailand, but also hopes that the western situation is changing.

The economic crisis is changing the closeness of Thai families and elderly people are being neglected. But western society is changing, I think, and western families are looking after their older people better, perhaps?

Finally, traditional Thai values of fun and accepting were noted:

Thais are different to western. Physically different and the way of living is different, more* sanuk *[fun] and more* mai pen lai *[it's no problem, don't worry].

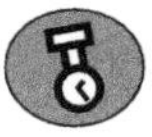

Communicating power

The hierarchy

As discussed earlier, Thai people are constantly assessing their position and status in relation to others. The informants in this study spoke of these relationships.

Big person/little person is a major issue. Thais always attempt to work out who is big and who is little. Sometimes, they are told by others, what that person's status is.

Degrees of seniority were also found in the student groups of nursing colleges.

In the nursing college, each year is 'senior to the previous', and students in each year must pay respect to the people in the year above.

Similarly, but less uniformly, patients have to find their position in the health-care and nursing hierarchy. This was the least clear area for the people interviewed. There was often a tension between the perceived, 'universal' nursing idea of 'treating everyone the same' and the problem of that person's status. The issue was further complicated by the nurse's own position in the health-care hierarchy. Patients may be either 'big' or 'little' according to their status outside hospital.

The big person/little person role is played out in hospitals, usually in line with rank or 'chain of command'. Patients may be either big or little, depending on their position. Sometimes patients who are little persons are treated the same as those who are big persons. Nurses should treat everyone the same. But nurses can order people to do things, if the patient is a little person. The head nurse occupies a middle position in the hierarchy. Junior nurses are little persons, while doctors are often big persons. However, the head nurse can be treated as reasonably equal by doctors.

Sometimes, the status of patients, in terms of their age, was reflected in the way in which they were spoken to:

Nurses treat older patients respectfully, sometimes calling them "Uncle" or "Aunt". Older patients get more respect than younger ones.

This informal, 'respectful' addressing of patients seems different from the ways in which, in the past, nursing in the west might address patients as 'Dear' or 'Love'. The terms 'Uncle' and 'Aunt' do not appear to suggest patronisation on the part of nurses or doctors.

Question for reflection

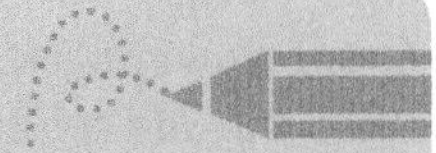

What do you think of a hierarchical system in hospitals, particularly one where patients may be treated differently according to their status?

Buddhism

The national religion in Thailand is Buddhism, which clearly permeates all aspects of life, including nursing and health care. Symbolic representations of the Buddha, in the form of statues, play a large part in the process of observing Buddhist worship. In health and illness, Buddhism plays an important role.

Sometimes we go to a Buddhist image and make pledge to give money after the person is well again. This is a form of **merit making.** ***We usually have a Buddha image in our homes, too. Buddha images are never bought: they are always only 'on loan'.***

Some participants also maintained that worship and the presence of family members may help to restore the patient's *Kwan* [life spirit] (it is also worth noting that in Thailand the words *Kwan* and *Khwan* are used interchangeably but mean the same thing). They therefore felt that providing patients with the opportunity to worship and an open visiting policy might help them to recover.

I am planning that every patient who is admitted to the ward is taken to a Buddha image or an image of the King, to worship [the King] who is the 'owner' of this hospital and the patients will tell him this, and this will help **khwan** ***to come back. My ward is an open one. Relatives can stay 24 hours and sleep in chairs by the beds.*** **Khwan** ***will come back if relatives are with the patients.***

This head nurse was clearly helping her patients to 'make merit', an issue discussed in more detail in the next section. Her reference to '*kwan* coming back' is also discussed at various points in this report. *Kwan*, the 'life spirit', can leave a person's body in illness or shock. The head nurse was helping patients to make sure that *kwan* came back by encouraging them to have their relatives with them.

Merit making

Merit making is the system of doing good in order to help redress the balance of one's own, possibly bad, karma, or to help the positive balance of karma for another person. A person might make merit on behalf of a sick relative. Flowers were used to help make merit for patients, usually in the form of a small garland of jasmine and rose flowers.

These garlands could be seen hanging over the beds of patients in the hospital.

Most of the nurses interviewed in this study were of the view that nursing itself was merit making.

Nursing is merit making? The most in the world. I was born to be a nurse. My husband is a doctor and I am a nurse, probably because we worked hard in a previous life.

Many nurses and relatives did go to the temple to make merit.

Reasons for going to wat [temple] are: to reduce karma, for fortune telling and to make merit.

The links between merit making, karma and illness were sometimes made explicit.

Thais believe that illness is caused by karma. I do myself. Thais make merit after illnesses to make positive karma.

Sometimes, Thai reticence seemed to be at work when talking about karma and merit making and other Buddhist notions. Nurses are likely to feel that illnesses are a result of bad karma. Given that nursing is viewed as a form of merit making, nurses will be anxious to help look after their patients. Serious illnesses, such as cancer, are more likely to be attributed to bad karma from either the present life or a previous one. Some head nurses will make arrangements for patients to make merit by offering food to monks or visiting a local shrine or statue of Buddha. In the following extract, an informant at first denies the notion of karmic influences in illness . . .

Is illness caused by karma? No. Some people think so - lower, less educated people. Although, sometimes, I do too.

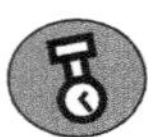

Male domination

Male domination in Thailand is widely written about in the press. Although there is a women's movement, the sticking point for some is the Sankha, or the community of Buddhist monks. Although there are

Buddhist nuns in Thailand, they are not perceived as having the same status as monks.

Perhaps because of this male domination and because of a (sometimes) clear distinction between male and female roles, nursing was not generally perceived as being suitable work for a man.

I asked a male nurse, "Did you get teased?" "Yes, I did, but I don't care. I have a girlfriend." He was being teased about being homosexual.

It is interesting that, first, it is widely unacceptable to have men in nursing, and second, that if men do go into nursing, they are likely to be thought of as being homosexual. Male nurses in the UK were also often once thought to be probably homosexual, and it is difficult to trace the reasons for this, although it is perhaps associated with the fact that the profession has traditionally been dominated by women. Also, in the Thai context, it is notable that in the 19th century, before westernised medicine was widely used in Thailand, it was the monks (male) who cared for the sick.

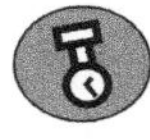

Kwan

Kwan is the 'life spirit' or 'power inside' that is sometimes thought to enter the body through the top of the head during birth. Many feel that '*kwan* goes away' (or is reduced) when a person is ill (including mental illness) or has had an accident. There are a variety of ways that Thais believe that a person's *kwan* can be restored. For example, when people return to their villages after a long journey, a *kwan* ceremony will often be performed by an elderly, female member of the community. In this ceremony, pieces of string that have been blessed at the temple are tied around the wrist, to 'bind the *kwan* to the body'. Similar ceremonies are performed by monks in various temples.

Relatives will engage in merit making to encourage **khwan** ***to come back. Flowers in garlands also help kwan to come back.***

Others, especially the younger participants, were more sceptical, although it was always difficult to know the degree to which people were reticent to acknowledge that they believed in the notion, as was sometimes the case when discussing karma.

My generation does not believe in* kwan*, but older people do. They believe that when people are sick, their* kwan *leaves the body. Younger people do not believe this so much.

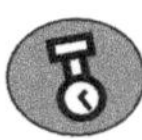

Communicating health and illness

Thai doctors

To the average Thai person, the doctor has senior status. Consultation time with a doctor averages about two minutes, so medical decision making is quick and diagnoses are made quickly. To fully appreciate what a doctor is saying requires at least a minimal understanding of the concept of 'medicine' and also of pathology. Clearly, many Thai people will have neither, nor will they be prepared to ask questions or challenge the doctor.

Patients trust doctors more than nurses. They are higher status and have more information. Most diagnoses are sound, but sometimes the consultation is too quick and mistakes are made. The average consultation time is two minutes. Patients are too shy to ask, if they do not understand.

Traditional medicine

Respondents maintained that some patients preferred traditional Thai medicine as a first choice in illness. Some of the interviewees also noted that they used **traditional medicine** for 'prevention' rather than for treatment.

Traditional Thai medicine is an oral tradition, passed on by people telling each other about it. We must keep this. Let the people help themselves. There was only the one traditional system in the past. Used without a research basis, but it would be good to make it more mainstream:

to do research into it. A lot more Thai people are using traditional Thai medicine for prevention. Not so much for cure, but sometimes for rehabilitation. We have lots of information now and it is starting to get researched. I had some back pain and I went to a modern hospital for treatment. It didn't work. Then I went to a traditional Thai medicine practitioner, who did massage, and it made me feel better.

Another informant noted the informal, family-based nature of the application of Thai medicine.

More people are going to traditional Thai medicine people for massage and things. When patients go home, they can call each other and ask each other to go to traditional healers. People with chronic illness want to get better quickly, so they go to traditional healers, looking for cures and hoping to get better quickly. Because of the characteristics of the Thai family they can all help the person to get better and pass on 'cures' to each other. Things they have learned over the years are passed on. It is an oral tradition.

The hospital

Going to hospital is rarely a pleasant or anxiety-free experience. For Thai people, especially those from outside the capital, there may be other associations: it is a place where people die, and therefore there may be bad spirits there. It is also a place where patients encounter people of a higher status, and where the usual forms of social interaction seem no longer valid.

In this study, there was evidence both of the things that may provoke anxiety and some of the means of reducing it. First, it was noted that nurses and other health professions do transgress the normal boundaries and taboos - for example, in being able to touch people's heads for treatment purposes. It was noted by some informants that older people in particular did not welcome this transgression. The patient who requires treatment or dressings to the head cannot say 'no' to the person who is offering them. In the first place, it would be rude and impolite to do so, and secondly, it is clearly necessary if the person is to recover their health. There is therefore a tension between the broken taboo and the need for it to be broken.

Respondents were more ambiguous about the degree to which they felt that patients occupied a lower status than nurses and doctors. However, it seems likely that, in a hierarchical society, 'submitting' yourself to the will of others (in the way that patients have to when they are admitted to hospital) is unlikely to be a pleasant experience. From having been in control as a member of their family and social group, the person suddenly finds themselves in a social grouping that is not of their choice. They have to relate to strangers as other patients, and to strangers who are inclined to tell them what to do (nurses, doctors and other health-care professionals). Thais are often quoted as being conservative and not particularly welcoming change. This factor is also likely to cause increased anxiety in the person who suddenly finds themself a patient in hospital.

Medicine, strong and quick

Thai people tend to like their medicine to be strong and to work quickly, and may be very disappointed if a visit to the doctor does not involve the issuing of a prescription. Local pharmacies, too, often given advice about medicines and, when asked, will offer a range of tablets to be taken simultaneously. A description of a cold may produce three different sorts of tablet for the customer to buy and take.

'Strong' medicine seems to be important. For a medicine to work, it is best if the patient feels something directly as a result. Many medicines, such as antibiotics, that are only available on prescription in other countries, are not regulated in this way in Thailand.

Communication and nurse education

Various training and education options are open to those who want to become a nurse in Thailand. These range from a 1-year practical nurse training course, through to a 4-year Registered Nurse course. A range of bachelor's, master's and PhD programmes are also available at various universities, including Thailand's most prestigious and oldest, Chulalongkorn, in Bangkok.

Students and teachers

In Thai schools and colleges - and in nurse education - teachers are highly respected and often viewed as *in loco parentis*, i.e. surrogate parents. It is not easy to get Thai students to challenge a teacher: what the teacher has to say is important, and to challenge them, and for the teacher to be wrong, would mean a loss of face for both parties.

For the western person, it therefore appears that much learning takes places by rote: students simply take down what the teacher says and later reproduce it in exams and papers. There is, of course, a long tradition of this form of 'oral learning'. Many of the great religious traditions rely on faithful transmission of 'the truth'. Sometimes, this faithfulness in teachers mystifies visiting teachers from the west, where there is the opposite tradition: in the west, students are encouraged to challenge what their teachers say and to engage in free and open debate with them.

Juethong (1998), in her study of Thai nursing students' relationships with their instructors, noted that those students wanted a caring relationship with their teachers, and hoped that the teachers would provide a home-like atmosphere in the school of nursing.

Students and teachers are close, and students respect their teachers. A '*Wai* Teacher's Day' is held every year, during which students pay respect and offer thanks to their teachers in a colourful and moving ceremony. Songs and poems are written and performed by the students. If scholarships and sponsorships are offered to students, they may be presented on this day. Following the more formal part of the ceremony, the students offer a concert to their teachers, ranging from stand-up comedy to classical Thai music rendition, dance and singing.

It is conceivable that a problem may arise out of this deep respect for teachers. Given the Thai reticence to challenge or question, teaching and learning often involve rote learning: students are not particularly required to be critical of what they learn, and would certainly not openly challenge what is taught. For example, even students taking higher degrees are unlikely to offer a particularly critical review of the previous literature, but more likely a summary of what has gone before.

It seems likely, too, that teachers enjoy the respect they get from their students. This attitude regarding the unquestioned knowledge of the teachers permeates the educational system, from early schooling to university. Further, according to reports from the informants and from column inches in national papers on the topic, Thai people do not read a great deal. Books are expensive and, presumably, reading is something of a solitary rather than a convivial activity (see also the next section). The question that arises is how the Thai knowledge base, in any discipline, can develop and grow. Klausner (1993) notes that there are no Thai 'philosophers' developing from the Thai universities, and suggests that university lecturers, having often studied abroad, quickly re-learn the prescribed role of university lecturers. That role seems to include the dispensation of information without its being questioned.

Question for reflection

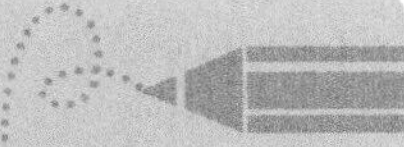

How does the educational system of rote learning in Thailand compare to your university education? Do you think there are any inherent problems in a university educational system where the students question little or nothing of their lecturers or existing empirical evidence?

To visiting academics from the west, who are used to 'knowledge being provisional' and always open to question, this comes as something of a shock. It is also slightly unnerving for the western academic to have their words treated with such reverence. In the west, university staff are used to the idea that the views they hold at one particular time may be replaced by others, as evidence from research or other sources (e.g. experience) supersedes them. Following, perhaps, from the unchanging truth of Buddhism, the knowledge available to Thai university staff seems to have a much longer shelf-life.

One other danger, perhaps, is that the 'west', in Thai terms, usually means the USA. Over the years, it would appear that academics from the USA have been quick to offer advice and information to their Thai colleagues, often in the form of consultancy work or as visiting lecturers. The information that comes out of the USA appears to be fairly unchanged for local consumption in Thailand, although the Thai people usually seem to take what they need for their own use. However, much of the academic language used in the colleges does appear to derive from the USA, without a lot of modification.

Whether or not Thai colleges will adopt a more adventurous approach to the generation and development of knowledge remains to be seen. On the one hand, it seems important for Thailand not simply to adopt other countries' ways of doing things, and on the other it seems equally important that its own knowledge base, in all disciplines, should be constantly regenerated though critical research. For this to happen, it would seem that the current almost overwhelming respect for teachers shown by students will have to be sacrificed for a more challenging approach to teaching and learning. However, this would undoubtedly involve overturning a number of Thai cultural norms and traditions, including *kreng jai* [politeness to others]. Therefore, in order to gain, a great deal would also be lost.

Ultimately, it must be possible for both teachers and students to respect each other, but to be able to challenge each other's views. What is at stake here, though, is not the 'teacher as a person', but their ideas. It is not a matter of blanket respect for a teacher and their knowledge: it is finding ways of respecting the teacher as a person, and also being able to offer argued and considered points of view that are different.

Reading

Various informants agreed that Thai people do not read very much. The exact reason for this is unclear. Some participants, however, maintained that they are just not taught to be good readers, whereas others suggested that books are expensive. Student nurses are often either given passages to read or directed to particular sections of books. An informant offered this view:

I do not like reading myself. I do not read the newspaper, but I listen to the news on the radio.

This is perhaps in keeping with the idea that Thailand has an 'oral' culture in which much is transmitted through talking. A letter in the English-language paper *The Bangkok Post* argued that Thai people did not spend their free time reading, as might be the case in some western cultures, as this was too 'solitary' an activity. Instead, they preferred to be with friends and family.

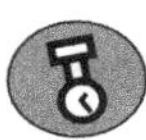

Nursing

Buddhism appeared to have an important influence on many aspects of nursing, and some of them are reported here. One respondent noted the ways in which Buddhism could help in care for the dying person.

Buddhist teaching can be applied to looking after dying people. Buddhism helps in the acceptance of dying, accepting pain. Pain must be accepted, but nurses and other health professionals, who have the means to alleviate pain, must also use those means.

Buddhism emphasises the need to accept that we age and die. Within the concept of *kreng jai* it is also important to accept pain when it occurs. However, to complain too much about pain would be to distress other people, and this would not be in keeping with *kreng jai*.

As we have noted, the hierarchical system of high and low also applies to the body, and this was noted in the nursing context.

Although the head is a high place and the feet are a low place, nurses have no problems with touching either of these for treatment. Sometimes, older people are concerned when nurses touch their heads.

In another context, the notion of high and low status was applied to the sort of care that might be expected and offered:

There are differences in treatment of VIPs and lower patients. There shouldn't be, but there are. VIPs get more visits from the doctor.

Similarly, student nurses sometimes felt low in status.

Thais speak quietly. They are shy, don't know what to ask, lack confidence, are unassertive, say "yes" when they don't understand. I often say to students: "Go to the doctor and ask him".

There is presumably the possibility of mistakes occurring as a result of this. If nurses tend to say 'yes', even when they do not understand, and not question what has been said, it seems likely that they may offer wrong information to patients or undertake inappropriate tasks. Similarly, patients may not understand what is being said to them by doctors, nurses and other health-care workers.

Question for reflection

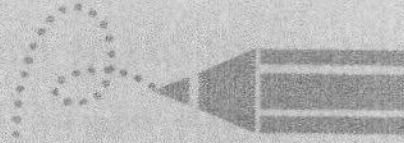

What do you think some of the potential problems are of nurses (qualified and students) saying yes, or nodding if they do not really understand what has been asked of them?

However, other respondents felt that communication between nurses and patients in Thailand was generally good, and therefore nurses should intervene in circumstances in which patients did not understand what the doctor had said.

Nurses should explain more about the illness and how patients can take care of themselves. The patients don't like to ask the doctor, so the nurses should ask for them and check if the patients have any problems or questions. Nurses also need more practice at getting information and

knowledge. It is changing with accreditation: nurses have to keep up to date.

However, doubts were often raised about the adequacy of some nurse-patient communication. Participants explained that communication between patients and nurses is often indirect and roundabout.

"Am I dying?" Make relatives happy and encourage a positive point of view, rather than saying "You are dying". Doctors are more direct, and senior ones are most direct of all, because of their status and knowledge.

According to that informant, then, doctors were perceived as more likely to have accurate knowledge, and because of this, and their status, they were also able to be more direct with patients. Another factor here is likely to be the short consultation time that doctors have with patients.

The Thai culture affects the way in which nurses talk, think and act. It's a circle. We do not have adequate communication because of the system, the hierarchy of the system. It is so slow to change. We have lots of one-way communication.

Given that nurses are likely to defer to doctors and patients defer to nurses, the reality of one-way communication seems likely. On the other hand, another informant offered a view of how this problem might be helped by time factors and by the Thai nurses' attitudes to patients and to care.

Western nurses work faster than Thai nurses because they just want to get the work done. Western nurses do not care about their relationship with patients. Thai nurses want better relationships with their patients. Thai nurses do not get angry with patients. We do not express anger. To be patient, to be calm. It is not polite to express emotion. We want to maintain **kreng jai.**

Again, though, this approach to nursing was deemed to be changing in Thailand, and some participants felt that younger nurses were now not so concerned with, for example, caring for relatives and simply wanted to 'just do their job'. One informant described a way in which she sought to overcome some of the possible communication problems between doctors, nurses and patients and to improve the quality of life for patients.

I have a board on my ward where patients can write how they feel about the doctors and nurses and treatment. They can either put their names there or not.

Communication in nursing

Thais typically speak quietly and often do not use non-verbal forms of communication in the same way as westerners do.

Thais use tones in their language to communicate, while westerners use more non-verbal communication and body language. Thais are taught to be quiet, polite and demure, and do not use their hands to communicate in the ways that westerners do.

One informant offered a challenge to the notion of the 'high-context culture', in which much was successfully communicated indirectly. In the following passage, the informant seems to suggest that such communication is not always so clear.

In Thailand, it is difficult to know what people really mean. There is always indirect communication. People are polite, but what are they really thinking? They often say, It's up to you! They have such a desire to please others.

Others pointed to the importance of teaching and learning communication skills in nursing colleges.

The Thai Nursing Council has set up competencies for nurses, and communication is one of the competencies. It is

one of the challenges for nurse teachers in Thailand, to teach good communication skills. Nurses are trained to be good communicators and to be mediators between doctors and patients. They need to be able to explain medical terms to patients and to translate what the doctor means.

Perhaps doctors in Thailand also need communication skills training? The short amount of time they spend with patients suggests that they may not have sufficient time to answer patients' queries properly - a factor likely to be complicated by the patient's reticence to ask questions.

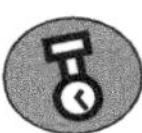

Other communication issues

From this study, Thai interpersonal communication in general can be characterised as follows. Face to face, Thai people will talk quietly and use limited eye contact, particularly across the sexes, or between two people who are not of equal status. Both parties will seek to maintain *kreng jai*, to make sure that each feels comfortable, and that neither party is compromised. **Turn-taking** between the two people is likely to be less marked than in many western cultures.

Communication and discussion are likely to be 'roundabout', rather than direct and to the point. It is sometimes better for a person to say what the other person wants to hear than to risk being controversial or confrontational. As a rule, confrontation and conflict are to be avoided. Gossip is likely to be a common feature of Thai communication, as is the use of compliments. In general, the aim is to ensure that both parties are respected and made to feel comfortable.

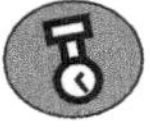

The Thai world view

The notion of Thai identity is an important one. Ekachai (2002) comments on how the persistence of beliefs in the supernatural (a fundamental part of Thai culture) shows how firmly traditions remain rooted in modern Thailand. She suggests that those beliefs are not edged out by consumerism but coexist very well. She also notes that the hierarchical structure of Thailand shows no sign of changing:

We may don modern clothes and work in gleaming high-rises, but the unspoken code of conduct which determines how we must relate to others and who gets what is still deeply rooted in our culture, which is essentially hierarchical and is based on a personal network. ***(Ekachai, 2002)***

Thai people are thought to be deeply conservative by nature and prefer the well-ordered, predictable world which, albeit impermanent in Buddhist terms, does not change too quickly and by so doing, cause them anxiety. Suwanna (quoted by Ekachai, 2002) notes:

Any society whose cosmos is based on the principles of non-permanence, subjection to suffering, and non-self faces a difficulty in explaining what reality is and how we explain the meaning of our lives. ***(Ekachai, 2002)***

Most Thais would probably prefer not to address that impermanence and suffering head-on, but to accept it and accommodate it by steering around it, by speaking softly and by having thought for others. For, in the end, others are suffering too.

In attempting to identify the Thai world view, Satha-anand and Bunyanetr (as cited in Ekachai, 2002) asked prominent Thai academics to identify words that they felt characterised Thai society. From their study, they noted that the 'Thai cosmic order' is characterised by words such as *chaat phop* (lifetimes), *phrom likit* (fate), *chok* (luck), *phee* (supernatural powers and spirits), *kam* (karma, action in previous lifetimes), *sawan* and *narok* (heaven and hell).

Most notable about this list of characteristics is that they all point to things which are completely outside the immediate control of the individual. We can attempt to influence them (e.g. by our actions or by merit making) but we cannot control them directly. Nor, presumably, can we know whether our attempts to influence them have been successful. We can only do our best and avoid anything that might otherwise upset these influencing factors.

Also, considerable dependence on others leads to care in maintaining good relationships. In Thailand, it is important not to disrupt relations with others because you never know when you will need them. This, according to Suwanna (Ekachai, 2002), leads to the Thai preoccupation with avoiding conflict and confrontation. Changes are also difficult because one must take care not to betray one's group or the group's network. It is perhaps for this reason that the Thai family and 'close friends' grouping is so prominent. Outsiders presumably represent a potential threat to the stability that these relationships offer. Given that it is 'others' or 'me and the group' that are important, and not 'me' or 'the self', to maintain the group is to maintain one's sense of identity.

Suwanna (Ekachai, 2002) notes some of these tensions and the potential anxiety they can cause. She suggests that, as a result, the Thais have come to rely on certain safety valves - ways of safely reducing tension. Working as a release, she explains, are the Thai obsessions with ***sanuk*** (fun), *len* (playfulness or not being too serious), and the forgiving nature of ***mai pen rai*** ('its no problem; it doesn't matter'). She notes that:

These reactions to strict tradition can be seen as forms of Thai wisdom. Without them, we might have long ago gone insane.

The famous 'Thai smile' may also be a way of preventing conflict and of - literally - 'keeping face'. The smile can also hide anxiety and be a powerful way of deflecting criticism and hostility.

Finally, Thai people have a strong sense of who they are: they have what might be described as a strongly embodied sense of self. Compared to western people, they usually appear to have a much more acute sense of their own bodies-in-space, and this contributes to the gracefulness of movement that can be noted on any day in any place in Thailand.

However, it is perhaps worth noting that one of the potential dangers of this type of cultural analysis is that of perceiving people as 'others'. Although it is difficult not to make comparisons between different sorts of people, it is also important not to single out groups of people only in terms of their differences. This sort of comparison can sometimes end up in a moral debate. Such, perhaps, was the thinking behind some missionary work: religious groups perceived groups of foreign people as 'others', and were determined to make them 'us'. Likewise, colonialism follows a similar path. Madrid (1994) makes the following comments about 'being other':

> ***Being the other is feeling different; it is awareness of being distinct; it is consciousness of being dissimilar. Otherness results in feeling excluded, closed out, precluded, even disdained and scorned . . . There is sometimes a darker side to otherness as well. The other disturbs, disquiets, discomforts. It provokes distrust and suspicion. The other frightens, scares.*** *(Madrid, 1994)*

Interestingly, Thai socialisation means that Thai people are always striving not to be outsiders. Their concept of self perhaps depends very much on being part of the group. In the first instance that group is a family one, but it soon extends to the friendship group, which includes both fair-weather friends and close friends. Although the Buddhist notion of non-attachment extends to friendships and even love affairs, Thai people generally want to be part of a friendship group. However, in doing so, they accept that friends come and go. There is not the urgency to be attached to friends or even lovers in the way that can exist in western countries.

However, it is not particularly useful to attempt to suggest that 'we are all the same under the skin', as if the differences we observe are not important: they are, and cultural sensitivity demands that we open our eyes to them and have some kind of awareness and respect for other people's beliefs and traditions.

We often adapt to a different culture, particularly if we spend a long time in that culture. However, adapting to a culture is one thing and 'becoming Thai' is quite another. The anthropologist Niels Mulder (2000) spent 5 years in Thailand, and left saying that he felt he had not made one close friend. Fitting into a culture and being able to throw off your own enculturation seems, perhaps, an unlikely enterprise. In

Thailand at least it would seem that those from other countries are always, to varying degrees, outsiders. To be Thai is to be born Thai, of Thai parents, and to have been socialised in the Thai culture. Arguably, no westerner coming to live in Thailand, for however long, is going to qualify on these points.

However, things are of course changing all the time, even in Thailand. Globalisation means that many younger people are forgetting some of their Thai socialisation and turning instead to other values and behaviours, most notably from the west. Globalisation is the global movement of western (usually North American) ideas and values. There is little to see of Thai values and behaviours being adopted by western cultures (except perhaps its cuisine, and in the 'Buddhist' trinkets available in shops). What is being lost is not simply about western people considering ways of acting: it is about western people not considering other ways of thinking and being. For it is not simply surface behaviours that make up a culture, but a difference of value systems, of ways of being, of beliefs about relationships and the world.

Western globalisation may even mean a loss to the world of those cultural factors that could benefit others. Almost paradoxically, learning about other cultures often means to stand aside and consider one's own. Ingrained ideas and beliefs often have to be set aside in order to appreciate that there are other ways of thinking, believing, feeling and doing. And, in a sense, this is what Thailand teaches you: to let go.

In summary - and borne out by the findings of this study - the factors that influence the Thai world view include the following:

- Being Thai by birth
- Speaking the Thai language
- Being a Buddhist and accepting Buddhist principles
- Incorporating aspects of spiritism alongside those Buddhist beliefs
- Respecting the hierarchy, including having complete respect for the monarchy
- Being polite, placatory, accepting of others, having fun and not being too serious.

Conclusion

This chapter has provided an overview of an ethnographic study exploring communication and culture in Thailand and in Thai nursing and health care. It is to be hoped that it has provided some food for thought, by comparing and contrasting cultural similarities and differences. The next chapter explores issues relating to studying and exploring cultural issues.

Suggested reading

Ekachai S (2001). *Keeping the Faith: Thai Buddhism and the Crossroads.* Bangkok: Post Books.

McClaren MC (1998). *Interpreting Cultural Differences: the Challenge of Intercultural Communication.* Derham: Peter Francis.

Mills L-J (1999). *Buddhism Explained.* Chiang Mai: Silkworm.

Mulder M (2000). *Inside Thai Society: Religion, Everyday Life, Change.* Chiang Mai: Silkworm.

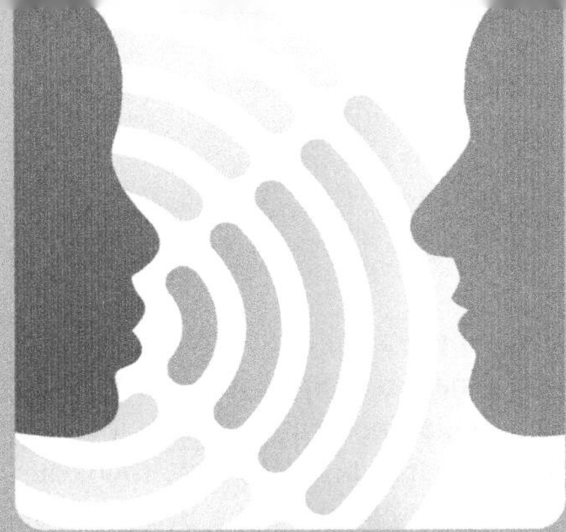

Chapter 5

Learning culture

Learning outcomes

At the end of this chapter, you should be able to:

- ✔ consider ways in which we develop our own cultural norms
- ✔ discuss methods of studying 'culture'
- ✔ identify the value and problems of ethnography as a means of studying cultural beliefs, values and associated issues

Introduction

This chapter explores how humans develop cultural norms, including beliefs and behaviours, and discusses how aspects of these cultural beliefs and behaviours can be observed and studied.

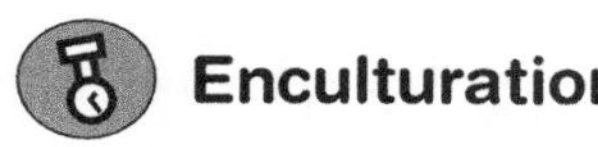

Enculturation

We learn about our culture from the moment we are born. Indeed, the process is known as enculturation (Barnard and Spencer, 2002). Being born into a particular culture at a particular moment in time is, it would seem, an accident and not of our choosing. In this sense, then, our being who we are is accidental: we do not choose to be British, Thai, North American or anything else. From day one, we are introduced to all of the norms and traditions of our own particular society. Our early days give us information about how children are brought up, how to behave with adults, how to treat school teachers and so on. Until we are old enough to reflect on what we are learning, we have no choice but to accept what we are taught or how we are socialised. This moment of realisation - that we do not *have* to believe what we are taught, and we do not have to believe that everything *has* to be this way - is sometimes known as the **existential moment**.

Many of us can probably remember when we first realised that we could think for ourselves. However, by then, the socialisation and enculturation process has arguably become so deeply embedded in who we are that we cannot change fundamental aspects about ourselves, even if we want to. We can, though, change a whole range of things about ourselves. For example, we can change or dismiss our religion or our religious beliefs. The second author (PG) was brought up as a Christian in the UK, attended church regularly as a child, and was christened in a Church of England Church. However, as he got older, and particularly after studying anthropology at university (where the existence of God was not questioned, but where aspects of the degree raised personal questions about the fundamental human belief in the existence of some kind of 'higher being' - i.e. that as humans, we often cannot believe that this really is it) he began to question the existence of God. Although I would not class myself as an **atheist**, my view of God and religion has now changed beyond all recognition from the unquestioning child that I once was. This vignette is not intended to be a religious sermon, but is merely offered as a practical example of how a key aspect of one person's beliefs can, and often does, change over time, particularly with life experience and further education.

Furthermore, we can question that what we are taught at school is not necessarily true, and so on. The degree to which we do all this challenging, also depends on our culture. In western cultures, people are frequently challenged by their teachers to reflect critically on what they have been taught and on what they believe. In many eastern and Islamic cultures, this critical view is often not only not encouraged but may be positively discouraged.

Question for reflection

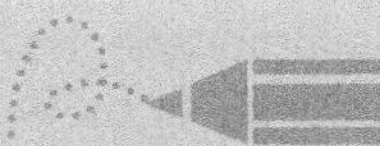

In the process of growing up, are there any things, such as beliefs or traditions (major or minor), that you have now subsequently questioned, modified or dismissed? For example, do you hold the same fundamental beliefs that you did five, 10 or even 15 years ago? If not, why did you change those beliefs? If so, why do you still believe them?

As discussed earlier in this book, one issue that most people are affected by is ethnocentricity: the tendency for us to believe that what we have learned about our own culture and ways of life is true, right and even superior, and that other cultures may therefore be wrong or inferior (Van der Geest, 1995). Given the discussion above, this is hardly surprising. We have, since birth, been learning all about one culture: our own (unless, of course, we have lived in a variety of different countries). However, as adults we should be able to reflect on what we know and make our own minds up. Nonetheless, it is perhaps worth pointing out that ethnocentricity, in its extreme form, is one of the major factors in human history that has contributed to persecution, conflict and even war (Lewis, 1985).

If all of this is true of us as individuals, it is also possibly true of many of the patients that we care for. Imagine a ward in which each bed is occupied by someone from a different country and a different culture. Each of those people is likely to believe that how they view the world is accurate and right. They are also likely to be either slightly surprised by the views of the people in surrounding beds, or to believe that those peoples' views are peculiar or simply wrong. Similarly, the nurses caring for this group of people are likely to have views on the peculiarity or rightness or wrongness of what their patients think, based partly on their own cultural beliefs. Bear this in mind when you are looking after people from other cultures. Like you, they have been 'acculturated' from birth. They believe that what they think about the world is accurate and largely true. Like you, if they did not believe this, they would probably change their minds and think other things. In believing a particular set of principles, we may believe that other principles are inappropriate or even wrong. We are, it seems, trapped by our own certainty about the world.

There is, however, an alternative to this, and that is to hold our ideas and beliefs about the world lightly. That is to say, we hold our set of views as provisional and open to change. In other words, we are prepared to change in the light of experience. Easy to say, but perhaps not so easy to do.

As we get older, we engage further in education: at primary, secondary and – for many – higher education levels. Much of what we are taught is culture bound. That is to say, the material is nearly always written by those from a similar culture and supports the culture in which that material is taught. Indeed, education can be defined, rightly or wrongly, as the passing on of the prevailing culture. However, increasingly throughout the world, where it is economically viable, students, particularly of university age, are being sent to study in other countries. This allows them a different view of culture – at least for anything from a few months to a few years. The problem that may occur is that, if and when those students return to their own culture, a number of things can happen: they are so changed by their experience in another culture that they cannot resettle in their own; they settle back into their own culture and re-establish their thinking in line with their original views; or they appreciate that there are other ways of looking at things, even if it has a minimal impact on their life. This is not a criticism but an **evaluation** of what often takes place. Whether or not it will ever be possible for any student to take a fully 'global' look at the world and absorb all of the various cultural viewpoints remains questionable. For example, finances aside, it is unlikely that one person will ever be able to visit every major region in the world, or even study or gain a meaningful insight into every culture in the world.

Case Study

Culture and nursing: an Australian nurse's perspective

I entered nursing at a time when there were few males, and when those males that worked in nursing were regarded as somewhat effeminate. Nevertheless, the early 1970s was a time of liberation, and Australian culture encouraged gender equality and equal opportunity. Our hospital, where I completed a 3-year certificate to become an RN, strongly encouraged male nurses. I must say that at the time my family, who expected me to complete a science degree of some type, were quite taken aback, yet supportive.

I'm not sure if I would be the same had I worked in nursing in another culture, but I do feel that the Australian culture that has influenced my development has been one of equality and being offered a 'fair go'; a culture of empowering professions previously heavily dominated by other professions or genders; and an enlightened government who believed in the professional development of nurses.

These cultural influences I have carried with me and have influenced my practice and work as an academic in several different cultures. In a nutshell, I believe I am confident, yet humbly aware of other cultures and their nursing practices; innovative yet patient, and a believer in time and consistency building credibility; open and democratic in my leadership style (to my detriment in some cultures); empathic and encouraging of colleagues who are disadvantaged by culture, economics or politics; and a believer in traditional scholarship and related ethical behaviour (again to my detriment in some foreign cultures).

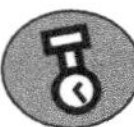

Methods of studying 'culture'

As discussed earlier, culture as a concept is difficult to define, and is arguably inextricably intertwined with a variety of other factors, psychosocial, historical and educational (Lewis, 1985). Consequently, culture itself probably cannot be studied in isolation, and is therefore usually explored by studying people from other (or even similar, depending on the research and the researcher) cultures, usually through the use of qualitative research methods.

Qualitative research aims to explore the behaviours, attitudes, beliefs, thoughts, feelings and views of other people (Silverman, 2000). The aim is not to generalise the findings but to offer a description of a particular setting at a particular time. Qualitative research is also often described as being 'naturalistic', in that it involves studying people in more natural environments, such as in their homes or at work (as opposed to an 'artificial' environment) (Parahoo, 2006). Methods of data collection used in such research vary, but commonly include interviews (individual or group interviews) and observations (including participant observations - where the researcher actively participates in activities with the participants - and non-participant observations, where the researcher merely observes practices, interactions and behaviour, without actively participating).

Holloway and Wheeler (1996) suggest that qualitative research contains the following elements:

- Qualitative research attempts to take the 'emic' perspective - the insider's point of view.
- Researchers immerse and involve themselves in the setting and the culture under study.
- The data have primacy: the theoretical framework is not predetermined by the data, but derives from it.
- The method includes 'thick description'.
- The relationship between the researcher and the researched is close and is based on a position of equality as human beings.
- Data collection and analysis interact.

In describing general ways of working within the qualitative framework, Parahoo (2006) observes the following:

In qualitative research, the methods of data collection, such as unstructured interviews and observations . . . are more

flexible and less structured. The questions are not always predetermined in advance nor are the same questions necessarily asked of all the respondents. Samples are not necessarily selected in advance of data collection. Researchers may decide to include or exclude respondents at any time during the research process. While the researcher can use props (such as notepads or tape-recorders) to record data, she may herself be a tool of data collection. Her mind records, registers and processes some of the information during interviews and observations as well as thereafter. Often she records some of the observations and thoughts in her diary as 'field notes'. *(Parahoo, 2006)*

As with any research approach, qualitative methods are not without their critics. Mays and Pope (1995) summarise some of the common criticisms:

The most commonly heard criticisms are, firstly, that qualitative research is merely an assembly of anecdotes and personal impressions, strongly subject to research bias; secondly, it is argued that qualitative research lacks reproducibility – the research is so personal to the researcher **(and also possibly the participants)** ***that there is no guarantee that a different researcher would not come to radically different conclusions; and finally, qualitative research is criticised for lacking generalisability.*** *(Mays and Pope, 1995)*

These points are hard to argue with, but in some ways they miss the point. To make these criticisms is, arguably, to argue from a quantitative perspective. Speaking from within the discipline of qualitative research, it is possible to accept the 'criticisms' but also to note that they are also part of the strengths of the approach. Qualitative studies do use anecdote and personal impressions – that is the point of them: to capture people's thoughts, feelings and beliefs. Qualitative research projects can rarely be replicated exactly, nor is it a researcher's intention that they should be. Different researchers, being human and bringing their own thoughts, feelings and beliefs to bear, would draw different conclusions and, as already noted, the aim of qualitative research is not to offer generalisable conclusions but to discover, describe and illuminate.

Furthermore, participants' experiences are often unique, and their views and beliefs about those experiences may also change over time (Cutcliffe and McKenna, 1999). For example, when research participants discuss their experiences, they are essentially talking about their beliefs, views and experiences of a phenomenon at a certain point in time. Therefore, if the same study was repeated with different respondents, or even with the same people but at a different point in time, it is questionable whether the study findings would be consistently the same (Gill, 2006). Even if the findings were identical, similar, or completely different, the studies would not necessarily be any less valid, provided they had both been conducted rigorously. Consequently, reliability (repeatability) as a methodological concept is arguably not an essential element of qualitative research.

Unfortunately, the debate about quantitative and qualitative research approaches in nursing has become rather polarised in recent years, with claims being made in some circles that the only 'right' approach is through the use of qualitative methods.

Early ethnographic studies, in the discipline of anthropology, seemed to be carried out with little thought of 'method'. The ethnographer took themselves off to the chosen site of study, 'immersed' themselves in it, took detailed field notes, and later wrote the ethnography. Later, as qualitative methodology challenged quantitative studies, particularly in the regions of just how objective and value free knowledge and methods in qualitative research were, ethnographers began to favour the 'naturalistic' approach (Lewis, 1985). In simple terms, this meant observing things as they were naturally occurring, without any attempt to control the environment under study (Evans-Pritchard, 1962). The researcher would also either attempt to stay shadowy and neutral 'in the background', or, as was often the case (particularly in later 20th century ethnographies), would actively participate in many aspects of daily life.

At best, it was felt that the researcher was simply a recorder of what was happening. However, later debates focused on the inherent difficulty of this position (Barnard and Spencer, 2002). A researcher is nearly always selective about what they observe, and always views an environment through a particular pair of cultural, psychological and sociological 'goggles' (Kuper, 1996), and is no more 'value free' than the quantitative researcher's bank of methods. Further, the researcher always (to varying degrees at least) contributes too, and changes what they are part of (Hammersley and Atkinson, 2007), and this can be viewed as an advantage rather than a problem. Using reflexivity (reflecting on personal, relevant behaviour, actions and beliefs), and by carefully noting their own reactions and changing perceptions, the researcher can add considerably to the value of the study (Parahoo, 2006). No longer is it advantageous for the researcher to hide in the background. Instead, they are an actor, front of stage, among other actors.

Ethnography has been used in a number of nursing and health-care studies relating to perceptions of health and illness. Nichter (1993) used it to explore the illness experience. Weiss (1988) undertook an ethnographic study to explore the use of explanatory models of illness and the absorption of new illnesses. Nichter (1993) used an ethnographic approach to understanding perceptions prior to health promotion interventions. Other ethnographic studies include those that observed record keeping (Allen, 1998); explored the transition from student to qualified nurse (Holland, 1999); exposed ritualistic practices in an operating theatre (Macqueen, 1995); and investigated curtain positioning in a maternity ward (Burden, 1998).

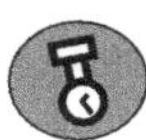

Evaluating ethnography

As already noted, the methods ethnographers (again, particularly anthropologists) have traditionally used can sometimes seem rather vague, although this is now less so, particularly in health-care settings. Field notes are usually written up after events have happened, and sometimes even after the researcher has left the field. Interviews must be transcribed, analysed and understood. Finally, a report is written (or, as is often the case, the report is written alongside the development of the study). As with all types of research, there must be ways of evaluating the quality of ethnographic studies (Hammersley and Atkinson, 2007).

Although there is much debate about how best to evaluate the quality of qualitative research (Cutcliffe and McKenna, 1999), Leininger (1991) offers the following criteria against which ethnographies might be evaluated:

- Credibility. Are the findings believable? Do they represent the 'real' world of the participants?
- Confirmability. Is all evidence documented and an audit trail established? Have member checks (checks with informants at the ends of the interview and study) been made?
- Meaning-in-context. Have informants been studied in context? Was account taken of their environment and the total situation?
- Recurrent patterning. Do the patterns which are uncovered recur and repeat themselves over time?
- Saturation. Did the researchers immerse themselves in the phenomena they have explored? Does the study show thick description? Has it gone so far that no further explanations and interpretations can be found?
- Transferability. Can the findings from this study be transferred to a similar context or situation under similar conditions? (Leininger, 1991).

It is perhaps worth pointing out that this list is by no means exhaustive, and there is a variety of other methods of assessing methodological rigour in qualitative research (Barbour, 2001). These issues are beyond the scope of this book, but if you would like to explore this area further, in more detail, please refer to the suggested reading list at the end of this chapter.

Nonetheless, Leininger's points, albeit useful, can be seen as open to criticism. The idea that patterns must recur and repeat themselves over time suggests a picture of a rather static culture (Helman, 2001). As discussed earlier, cultures are constantly changing. Similarly, it seems doubtful that any researcher would be able to 'go so far that no further explanations and interpretations [of the data] can be found'. Presumably, everything is always open to other explanations and interpretations. For example, a researcher may interpret the same data in different ways at separate points in time; or two or more researchers may interpret the same data differently (Gill, 2006). If their interpretations or analyses of the data are 'grounded' in those data, then neither is necessarily more right or more wrong than the other. But it does help to highlight the fact that data can always be interpreted differently. Suggesting otherwise would perhaps indicate that an objective view of the world is possible (Gill, 2006).

The issue of the relationship between culture and behaviour is a fraught one (Helman, 2001). The 'realist' ethnographers in the early 20th century often seemed to assume that describing behaviour was in many ways sufficient in the quest to describe culture. However, beyond and outside behaviour, people are meaning-makers: they construe their world and make sense of it through their own interpretations of it (Hendry, 2008). For this reason, it is not sufficient for a researcher merely to state: 'This is what I saw people doing'; it is also vital to ask people why they do what they do, and what meaning they ascribe to it. Failure to do so can result in misinterpretation by the researcher of the behaviour observed. Sometimes this meaning can be made explicit and sometimes not. For example, sometimes people are unreflective about what they do, or do not know why they are performing a certain action (Hammersley and Atkinson, 2007). Perhaps much of our lives are lived simply at the 'doing' level. Presumably, few people consider that what they do is 'part of their culture' - at least, not on a day-to-day basis.

Ethnography, as a research approach, is now being used increasingly in health-care settings, and often by researchers who are also health professionals, such as nurses and midwives (Hammersley and Atkinson, 2007). As in traditional ethnography, such research often combines methods of data collection such as participant observation and interviews. However, many health professionals who have undertaken empirical research (particularly in their own area or specialty) often find that research and clinical practice require two different types of 'hat': the researcher and the practitioner (Gill, 2006). Although the two roles share many similarities, they also have several fundamental differences, which can be especially problematic for novice health-care researchers. For example, nurses who conduct ethnographic research in their own area of clinical practice often find initially that they have been so immersed in that particular culture that they are to some extent blind to it. This is discussed further in the following case study.

Practice-based Case Study

Ethnographic research in midwifery practice

I am a practising midwife in a large teaching hospital in Wales, where I have worked for over 10 years. A few years ago I embarked on a PhD, exploring, among other things, interactions between midwives and parents during childbirth in the hospital delivery suite. The research was conducted using an ethnographic approach and I combined participant observation with in-depth interviews as my primary methods of data collection.

Some of the participant observations involved me actively participating in the delivery process, whereas others involved my simply observing practice and not actively participating unless required to do so (e.g. a medical emergency). My initial observations, however, were really quite superficial and I only ever seemed to collect observational data, which seemed to me to be relatively insignificant. I discussed this with my PhD supervisor (a male anthropologist, with no health-care qualifications), who also felt that my observations lacked any real insight, and we agreed that, provided we could find a family who were happy for him to be present, we would do some joint observations, to see whether we could identify any problems in the research process and establish a way forward.

We soon found a family who were happy for us both to be present at the birth of their child. We stayed in the delivery suite for several hours (although not continuously) and mainly observed, although we did actively interact with all present. We compiled field notes separately of the observations that we made throughout this process, and agreed that we would only discuss these issues after we had left the delivery suite.

Some time later, when we got together, we finally compared field notes. Again, my observations and notes were quite superficial, but my supervisor had made copious amounts of notes, with incredibly detailed and significant observations that I had simply been oblivious to. For example, the use of touch, issues relating to personal space, and non-verbal forms of communication between midwife, mother and father.

I was totally bewildered as to how he had noticed these things when I really hadn't, especially as it was my area of specialty. But when we spoke about it, he pointed out to me that he was viewing the birth, the interactions between all concerned and the delivery suite for the first time, with a 'fresh, objective pair of eyes', whereas for me it was a place where I worked on a daily basis and, consequently, I had paid little attention to the finer details of everyday practice.

I learnt a very important lesson that day. Ethnography, particularly when conducted in your own area of specialty, is often about making the familiar unfamiliar. As a researcher, it involves trying to look at things in a different way and questioning everything – for example, Why did they do that? What's going on there? On reflection, I had lost sight of the research agenda because I couldn't 'see the wood for the trees'. However, it is fair to say that when I went back to do further observations, I suddenly saw things in a different light. This incident, more than any other, made me realise that ethnography really is about opening your eyes to your environment.

The readers of an ethnographic study involving cultural issues are likely to be student nurses from various cultures, nurse educators, other researchers and academics (particularly anthropologists and other social scientists). However, in many ways the authors of an ethnographic report, or any written publication for that matter, can exercise little or no control over what the reader makes of the text, nor how they understand or interpret it. In this sense, the authors agree to some extent with the postmodern view that 'the reader writes the text'. Once a writer has committed their ideas to paper, there is nothing that can be done to persuade the reader that 'this is what I meant and I did not mean that'. The reader always brings to a text their own background, culture, belief system, opinions and a range of other factors, which means their reading is highly particular. It is probably a myth to believe that there are clear and transparent ways of reporting that are going to be unambiguous. However, it is perhaps especially important that writing, at all levels and for any audience, should be simple and clear

(Burnard, 2004). Although jargon can sometimes be used as shorthand to convey a set of reasonably well understood concepts, it is also a shortcut to misunderstandings and to negative judgements by readers. To paraphrase Wittgenstein (1966): 'That which can be said, can be said clearly. That of which we cannot speak, we should pass over in silence.'

Conclusion

This chapter has explored key issues relating to the process of enculturation, how aspects of cultural beliefs and behaviour can be observed and researched, and the use of ethnography as a research approach, particularly in health care. The next chapter explores religion and human beliefs.

Suggested reading

Atkinson P, Delamont S, Coffey AJ et al. (eds) (2007). *Handbook of Ethnography*. London: Sage.

Hammersley M and Atkinson P (2007). *Ethnography: Principles in Practice*, 3rd edn. London: Routledge.

Holloway I and Todres L (2006). Ethnography. In: Gerrish K and Lacey A, eds. *The Research Process in Nursing*, 5th edn. Oxford: Blackwell, pp. 208–223.

O'Reilly K (2005). *Ethnographic Methods*. London: Routledge.

Pope C and Mays N (eds) (2006). *Qualitative Research in Healthcare*, 3rd edn. Chichester: WileyBlackwell.

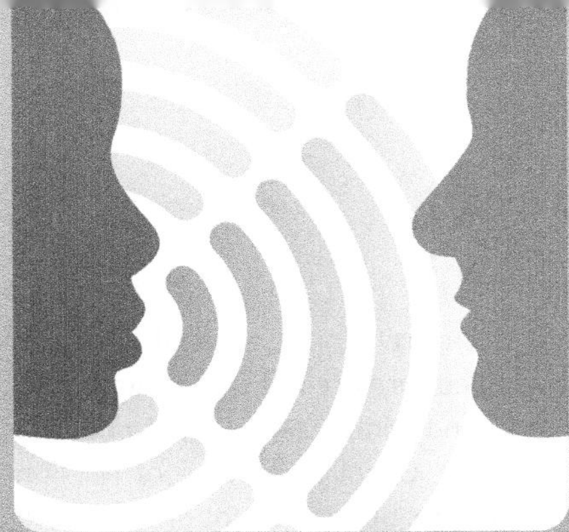

Chapter 6

Beliefs and religion

Learning outcomes

At the end of this chapter, you should be able to:

- ✔ consider your own religious beliefs, or lack of them
- ✔ identify some of the key concepts of major world religions
- ✔ discuss the importance of religion to the development of culture

Introduction

This chapter explores the impact of formal religion (focusing on the major religions) on culture and how religion can influence beliefs, behaviour and practice. It is intended to provide an overview of some of the key aspects of the major religions. For nursing students, it is hoped that this will provide insights into some of the more common religious beliefs. We do not offer a 'tick box' approach to the various religions, but hope that the chapter will provoke thought and allow appreciation of religions whose beliefs you may or may not share.

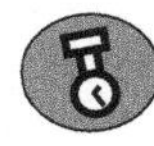

Religion

Behind most cultures will be found sets of religious beliefs. It is important to note, however, that religion and culture are not the same things. Religion, albeit in many cultures profoundly important, is just one of a variety of factors that can affect culture. Usually one type of religion dominates in a particular society or culture, but this is not always so. In the UK, for example, there is a mix of Christianity, Islam, other religious groups, agnosticism and unbelievers (these latter terms will be discussed later in this chapter).

In nursing, it is important to think about religion beyond the level of issues such as the diet someone should have, or whether or not to call the chaplain or Rabbi (although these are important issues too). It is also important to understand that many religious beliefs (or lack of them) are often inseparable from the way people live their lives (Bowker, 2006). They can affect everything from the ways in which people think about health, illness and treatment, to the way their families should or should not be involved in their care. They can also affect fundamental aspects of nursing, such as touch, dealing with gender, and beliefs and customs associated with death and dying (including organ transplantation). As nurses, we have a duty to learn all we can about the different major world religions, and also about the objections that some have to religious beliefs. Perhaps more than anything, we should neither assume that others believe the same things that we do, or that others *should* believe as we do.

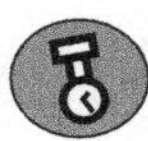

Respect

Before the main features of some of the world's major religions are considered, it is important to discuss some of the issues that arise when religion is discussed. First is respect for other religions. This can potentially be problematic. For example, if we firmly believe in a particular set of religious principles, we must theoretically also believe that they are 'true'. Consequently, if they are 'true', then other principles are, to some extent at least, false. Thus it seems unlikely that those who hold firm religious views (especially fundamental views, regardless of faith) will really 'respect' other religions. The best we can do is to respect the fact that other people have different views from our own, or have no views on religion at all.

The issue is perhaps more one of respecting people rather than respecting their particular beliefs. It should also be noted that religions vary in the degree to which their members are expected to attempt to draw other people in. Certain religions claim that it is impossible to 'join' them: the issue is determined at birth (Bowker, 2006). Others (such as the Jehovah's Witness sect of Christianity) place great importance on their members attempting to convert others to their own particular beliefs. Still other religions make no claims to attempt to convert in this way: Buddhism is such a one. Buddhists do not attempt to convert others to their way of thinking (Gyatso, 2001).

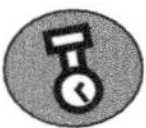

Belief and truth

A variation on the above point about truth is that religious beliefs cannot claim to be 'truths', in the sense that, say, the proposition $2 + 2 = 4$ is true. Religious beliefs are just that: beliefs, in that all major religions are founded largely on the principle of faith, i.e. they cannot be scientifically proved or, for that matter, disproved. Most people who hold religious beliefs also hold them to be true, but it is worth thinking for some time about this. There are various spoof 'religions' developing on the internet that highlight this issue. One is the 'religion' which has the 'Invisible Pink Unicorn' as its head. For more details, see: http://en.wikipedia.org/wiki/Invisible_Pink_Unicorn. It is claimed that the religion is based on both truth and belief. The unicorn is invisible, so that is the truth element, but it is also *believed* to be pink. The spoof is an attempt to highlight the problems that religions have with proving the existence of God. Many arguments in religion seem to focus on 'what God has in mind', although the existence of God is rarely questioned by believers. If it is impossible to prove the existence of God, then it is clearly also impossible to know what God has in mind.

In a number of religions there are at least two approaches to understanding what God requires or wants of people (Smart, 1998). The first is by reference to sacred texts (e.g. the Holy Bible or the Qu'ran). The second is by reference to 'revelation'. Christians need not confuse this issue with the Book of Revelation, in the Bible. Revelation, in the sense used here, means that God 'allows' us to understand things by gradually 'revealing' them to us.

In the case of sacred texts, opinions vary in the degree to which different sects believe that everything in a sacred text is a true reflection of God's 'mind' (Bowker, 2006). Some sects believe that those texts are the absolute word of God, and that everything written in them comes directly from God. Others believe that some or all of the texts are 'stories' that were handed down prior to written language. For example, evangelical Christians will tend to believe that the Bible is the absolute and irrefutable Word of God, and that its meaning is to be taken literately (Seaman and Brown, 1999). Some parts of the Church of England, however, might argue that what is read in the Bible is a set of stories about how people should live together and worship God. For Muslims, the Qu'ran - in the original language - is the absolute Word of God and cannot be modified or changed.

However, written words are often interpreted differently by different people, and this is particularly the case with both the Bible and the Qu'ran. It is perhaps also fair to say that over the years since both books were originally written, they have each undergone multiple interpretations. Of course, when discussing religions one must consider which interpretation of the written word is correct. In many religions this has caused a variety of problems, as there is no way of asking the original author(s) what they really meant. It is therefore up to the reader to decide, and consequently it is perhaps understandable how ambiguous text in particular, can be interpreted in a number of different ways.

Question for reflection

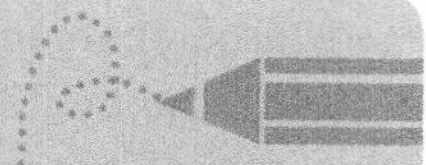

What are your own beliefs about religious issues? Could you say clearly to another person what you do or do not believe?

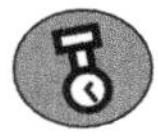

Agnosticism and atheism

The term **agnostic** tends to be used in two ways: a general way and a more precise way. The general use of the term is usually used to describe a person who does not have a particular set of religious beliefs and may or may not be open minded about whether or not God exists (Bowker, 2006). Such a person says they simply 'do not know'. A more strict meaning of the word is when it is used to describe a person who believes that, in the absence of proof of the existence of God, discussion on the matter is a waste of time. For this type of agnostic, it is not only impossible to know whether God exists, there is little value to be had in debating the issue. Particularly in the west a person will often say they are agnostic in order to indicate that they have not yet made their mind up about religion and about God.

Atheism is the positive belief that God does not exist (Bowker, 2006). This is moving beyond the argument that the existence of God cannot be proved or disproved, but that there is no such thing as 'God'. Some atheists follow the implications of this point of view through and argue that religions of all sorts are bad for society and for the world. Perhaps the best-known of those who argue in this way is the British professor and writer Richard Dawkins (2006), who published a controversial book called *The God Delusion*. In a similar vein, the North American writer Sam Harris (2006) published another book called *The End of Faith*, and Christopher Hitchens (2006) also published a similar book called *God is not Great: The case against religion*.

In the 1960s the British anthropologist Sir E.E. Evans-Pritchard (1966) published a book entitled *Theories of Primitive Religion*, where he explored the theory that religion could be a man-made concept which, among other things, served an important sociological and psychological function (e.g. the ordering of society). However, Evans-Pritchard's work was essentially the exact opposite of the books published by Dawkins et al., in that Evans-Pritchard was a born-again Christian (this apparently occurred during his earlier fieldwork in Africa). He therefore sought to prove the folly of such theories.

Unbeliever

The term **unbeliever** is perhaps a somewhat softer term for atheist and may sometimes refers to another sort of person. In essence, an unbeliever is one who does not believe in a God or in anything to do with the supernatural. The word 'supernatural' refers to the area of beliefs about what does or does not exist outside the physical world. For example, the earth clearly 'exists' in the physical world, as do tables, papers, books and computers. However, when we move into discussions of God, spirits, souls and other such things, we move into the domain of the supernatural - a domain beyond what can be seen, touched, tasted, heard or smelt. The unbeliever, when asked what exists outside the physical world, would answer 'nothing'. This is slightly, but not significantly, different from the atheist, who, while probably agreeing with the unbeliever, is really relating his disbelief specifically towards the non-existence of God.

Obviously, the problem with any notions of a world outside the physical is one of proof. If we cannot encounter things through our senses (taste, touch, smell, sight or hearing), how do we 'know' they are there? There is not space in a book of this type to go into the details of these debates, but the interested reader should consider studying them in greater depth.

Spirituality

In recent years, the term **spirituality** has been widely used in nursing (McSherry *et al.*, 2004), whereby nurses are expected to consider a patient's spiritual needs and respect them. The term spirituality, however, is not very well defined. In western literature it is often associated with religion, but it is just as likely to be linked to 'New Age' beliefs and things such as a belief in a 'power greater than ourselves'. Exactly how such a power differs from God is not usually well described.

Question for reflection

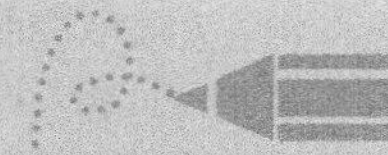

How would you define the word 'spirituality'? How can thinking about spirituality help the patients in your care?

On not having a religion

Before encountering a brief review of the main points of belief of some of the world's major religions, it is worth noting that many people in eastern countries are likely to find the idea of having no religion far more strange than having a different religion. Thus, to a Muslim, being a Christian may be acceptable, but having no religion at all is confusing.

A disclaimer

This chapter attempts, as far as possible, to represent some of the main beliefs and facts of the world's religions. Its purpose is to provide a brief overview of some of the key aspects of each religion, which are given in alphabetical order. We are not theologians, and many individuals and groups have different views on the finer points of a particular religion. We apologise in advance if we have made any mistakes in our summaries, and would urge the reader who wants to know more to consult the books recommended at the end of the chapter. Another good idea is to talk to people of various religions and see what they believe. You may find that their belief systems differ from more formal, more academic accounts.

Buddhism

Buddhism is a spiritual tradition that focuses on freeing people of the notion of 'self' and the attainment of a deep insight into the true nature of life (Bowker, 2006). Buddhism teaches that all life is interconnected, so compassion is natural and important – compassion for both people and all sentient beings. It is important to note that the Buddha was a man (some say one of many Buddhas) and not a god. Buddha, then, is not worshipped as such. Buddhism is 2500 years old and currently has 376 million followers worldwide. It is prevalent in many parts of South-east Asia, including Thailand, India, and parts of China and Japan. There are around 151 816 Buddhists in the UK, according to the 2001 census. Buddhism arose as a result of Siddhartha Gautama's quest for enlightenment in around the 6th century BC (Harvey, 1990). There is no belief in a god, although in some forms of Buddhism there is discussion of heavens and hells (Mills, 1999).

Buddhists believe that nothing is fixed or permanent: change is inevitable. The two main Buddhist sects are Theravada and Mahayana, but there are many more. Buddhism is a religion with many festivals throughout the year. Buddhists can worship both at home or at a temple. The path to enlightenment is through the practice and development of morality, meditation and wisdom and is developed by observing the **Four Noble Truths** and the Eightfold Path (Gyatso, 2001). Although translations of the Four Noble Truths, from ancient documents, can vary, they are often described as follows:

1. All life is suffering.
2. Suffering is caused by attachment (to things and people).
3. There is a way of escaping from suffering.
4. The way of escaping from suffering is by following the Eightfold Path.

In turn, the Eightfold Path offers a prescription for living and involves the following:

1. Right view
2. Right intention
3. Right speech
4. Right action
5. Right livelihood
6. Right effort
7. Right mindfulness
8. Right concentration.

The code of the Eightfold Path is thus both a moral one (or 'how we should live') and a practical one ('what we can do to relieve suffering').

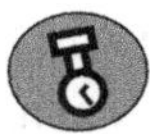

Christianity

Christianity is the most popular religion in the world, with over 2 billion adherents (Smart, 1998). In the UK, 42 million Britons see themselves as Christian, and there are 6 million who are actively practising. There are many different variations of Christian belief, including Catholicism. However, only the main tenets of Christianity are discussed here.

Christians believe that Jesus was the Messiah promised in the Old Testament, and they believe that Jesus Christ is the Son of God (Seaman and Brown, 1999). They also believe that God sent His son to earth to save humanity from the consequences of its sins.

One of the most important concepts in Christianity is that of Jesus giving his life on the Cross (the Crucifixion) to save the world, and rising from the dead on the third day (the Resurrection). Christians believe that there is only one God, but that there are three elements to this one God: God the Father, God the Son, and God the Holy Spirit (Seaman and Brown, 1999). Together, these are known as the Trinity, a concept not always easy to understand or to explain.

Christians worship in churches and their spiritual leaders are called priests or ministers. The Christian holy book is the Bible, which consists of the Old and New Testaments. Christian holy days such as Easter (the Crucifixion and the Resurrection of Christ) and Christmas (the birth of Christ) are important milestones in the Christian calendar.

Case Study

A UK teenager's account of Christianity

Christians believe in an omnipotent, omniscient, just and perfect God. This God created the world and everything in it. God then made humans to maintain his world, and to have a perfect relationship with him as king. Humans decided that they wanted to be king over their own lives, and went their own way. The Bible calls going our own way, away from God. Because God is perfect he cannot stand to be in the presence of sin, so when people went their own way they shattered the perfect relationship with God.

God is just and perfect, so He can't let sin go unpunished. So for thousands of years God's people had to sacrifice animals to take the punishment for sin instead of themselves. The problem with this was that people started sinning again and so needed more sacrifices. God saw that people were still getting things wrong, so he sent his son, Jesus Christ, to earth to be a sacrifice for

everyone. Jesus is God and was human at the same time. Because he was God he lived a perfect life, without sin, and taught people how he wanted us to live.

When he was 33 he gave his life as a perfect sacrifice for anyone and everyone who believes. Because he was a perfect sacrifice he outweighs any amount of sin that a person could do. This means that if someone accepts Jesus' sacrifice was for them and truly asks for forgiveness, then the punishment for their sins is taken on Jesus and they are made right in God's eyes. If someone accepts this as God's invitation to eternal life with him, then they are a Christian and will live with God for ever. If someone doesn't accept this invitation then they spend eternity cut off from God, which the Bible calls Hell.

Question for reflection

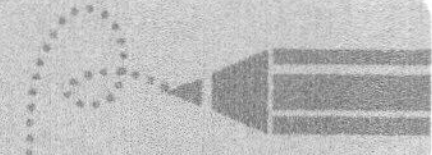

Many people in the UK if asked about their religion, may say that they are 'Christian'. If you feel you are a Christian, what does that mean to you? Does it mean you believe in the things described above? Do you go to church regularly? Or do you say you are Christian because you cannot think of anything else to say on the matter?

Hinduism

Hinduism is one of the world's oldest religions, and has over 900 million adherents worldwide (Bowker, 2006). Hinduism is not a single doctrine, and there is no single founder or teacher. Hinduism originated around the Indus Valley near the River Indus in modern-day Pakistan (Ganeri, 1999). About 80% of the Indian population regard themselves as Hindu.

Hindus believe in a universal eternal soul called Brahman, who created and is present in everything, but they worship other deities such as Ram, Shiva and Hanuman, recognising different attributes of Brahman in them (Ganeri, 1999). Hindus believe that existence is a cycle of birth, death and rebirth, governed by karma. Hindus believe that the soul passes through a cycle of successive lives, and its next incarnation is always dependent on how the previous life was lived.

The Vedas are the most ancient religious Hindu text and define the truth. Hindus believe that the texts were received by scholars directly from God and passed on for generations by word of mouth. Hindus celebrate many holy days, but Diwali, the Festival of Lights is the most well known. The 2001 census recorded 559 000 Hindus in the UK - around 1% of the population. It should be noted that it is probable that Buddhism grew out of Hinduism, and some of its concepts (such as that of being reborn into a different life, after death) have been incorporated into Buddhism.

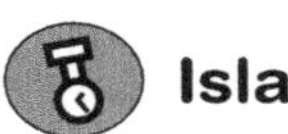

Islam

The word Islam means both 'peace' and 'submission'. It is the second largest religion in the world, with over 1 billion followers (Bowker, 2006). It was revealed over 1400 years ago in Mecca, Arabia. Followers of Islam are called Muslims. Islam is commonly practised in countries in the Middle East, North Africa and South-east Asia. The 2001 census recorded 1 591 000 Muslims in the UK, around 2.7% of the population.

There are several different groups of Muslims, but all of them, in every country and community, regard their faith as a bond between them, and as a major part of their identity (Weston *et al.*, 2005).

Muslims believe that there is only one God. The Arabic word for God is *Allah*. According to Muslims, God sent a number of prophets to mankind to teach them how to live according to His law. Jesus, Moses and Abraham are respected as prophets of God. They believe that the final Prophet was Muhammad. Muslims believe that Islam has always existed, but for practical purposes date their religion from the time of the migration of Muhammad (Weston *et al.*, 2005).

Muslims base their laws on their holy book the Qur'an, and the Sunnah. The Sunnah is the practical example of Prophet Muhammad. There are five basic Pillars of Islam. These are the declaration of faith, praying five times a day, giving money to charity, fasting, and (at least) a once in a lifetime pilgrimage to Mecca (Smart, 1998, Bowker, 2006).

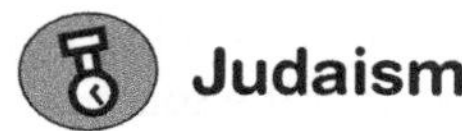

Judaism

Judaism is the original of the three Abrahamic faiths (after Abraham, in the Old Testament of the Bible), which also include Christianity and Islam. There are 12 million Jewish people in the world, most of them in the USA and Israel (Smart, 1998). According to the 2001 census, 267 000 people in the UK said that their religious identity was Jewish, about 0.5% of the population.

Judaism originated in the Middle East over 3500 years ago. It was founded by Moses, although Jews trace their history back to Abraham. Jews believe that there is only one God, with whom they have a covenant. In exchange for all the good that God has done for them, Jewish people keep God's laws and try to bring holiness into every aspect of their lives (Bowker, 2006). Judaism has a rich history of religious text, but the central and most important religious document is the *Torah*.

Spiritual leaders are called Rabbis and Jews worship in synagogues. It is estimated that 6 million Jews were murdered in the Holocaust in the Second World War (mainly by the Nazis) in an attempt to wipe out Judaism. There are many people who identify themselves as Jewish without necessarily believing in, or observing, any Jewish law.

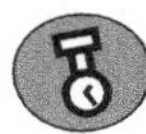

Sikhism

There are 20 million Sikhs in the world, most of whom live in the Punjab province of India (Bowker, 2006). The 2001 census recorded 336 000 Sikhs in the UK. Sikhism was founded in the 16th century in the Punjab district of what is now India and Pakistan. It was founded by Guru Nanak and is based on his teachings, and those of the nine Sikh gurus who followed him (Smart, 1998, Bowker, 2006).

The most important thing in Sikhism is the internal religious state of the individual. Sikhism is a monotheistic religion (the belief in the existence of one deity, or in the oneness of God) that stresses the importance of doing good actions rather than merely carrying out rituals. Sikhs believe that the way to lead a good life is to keep God in heart and mind at all times; live honestly and work hard; treat everyone equally; be generous to the less fortunate; serve others (Smart, 1998).

The Sikh place of worship is called a Gurdwara and the Sikh scripture is a book called the *Guru Granth Sahib*. The tenth Sikh Guru decreed that after his death the spiritual guide of the Sikhs would be the teachings contained in that book, so it now has the status of a Guru, and Sikhs show it the respect they would give to a human Guru (Bowker, 2006).

The community of men and women who have been initiated into the Sikh faith is the Khalsa. The Khalsa celebrated its 300th anniversary in 1999. Guru Gobind Singh decreed that where Sikhs could not find answers in the Guru Granth Sahib, they should decide issues as a community, based on the principles of their scripture (Smart, 1998).

Question for reflection

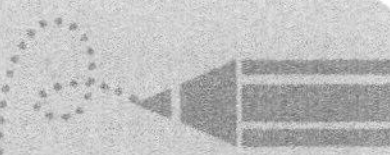

Many people, even those who deny that they are in any usual way 'religious', say that they 'believe in a power greater than themselves'. What do you think they might mean by this? Is it a belief that you have?

Unitarianism

There are about 7000 Unitarians in the UK and Ireland, and about 150 Unitarian ministers. There are about 800 000 Unitarians worldwide. Unitarianism is an open-minded and individualistic approach to religion that gives scope for a very wide range of beliefs and doubts. Religious freedom for each individual is at the heart of Unitarianism. Everyone is free to search for meaning in life in a responsible way, and to reach their own conclusions.

In line with their approach to religious truth, Unitarians see diversity and pluralism as valuable rather than threatening (Bowker, 2006). They want religion to be broad, inclusive, and tolerant. Unitarianism can therefore include people who are Christian, Jewish, Buddhist, Pagan and Atheist. Unitarianism has no standard set of beliefs. Unitarians believe that religious truth is not necessarily or primarily laid down either in scriptures, by a holy person or by a religious institution. No individual or group in Unitarianism makes an exclusive claim to the truth. Within certain core values each Unitarian can believe what they feel is right. Unitarians are so called because they insist on the oneness of God and because they affirm the essential unity of humankind and of creation (Bowker, 2006).

Unitarians believe religion should make a difference to the world, so they are often active in social justice and community work. Unitarianism grew out of the Protestant Reformation of the 16th century and started in Poland and Transylvania in the 1560s (Smart, 1998). Unitarians have adopted the Flaming Chalice as the symbol of their faith. The Unitarians were the first church in the UK to accept women as ministers, in 1904. Unitarians welcome gays and lesbians in their ministry, and support equal rights for gay and lesbian people within the Church and in society at large.

Conclusion

This chapter has explored some of the key elements of the world's major religions and some of the fundamental aspects of opposing views (for example atheism). Again, it is worth reiterating that this chapter is not intended to be a definitive guide to religion, and we would recommend that the reader who wishes to know more about such issues explore some of the books in the suggested reading list. The next chapter explores culture and cultural issues in nursing.

Suggested reading

Bowker J (2006). *World Religions*. London: Dorling Kindersley.

Dawkins R (2006). *The God Delusion*. London: Black Swan.

Evans-Pritchard EE (1966). *Theories of Primitive Religion*. Oxford: Oxford University Press.

Smart N (1998). *The World's Religions*, 2nd edn. Cambridge : Cambridge University Press.

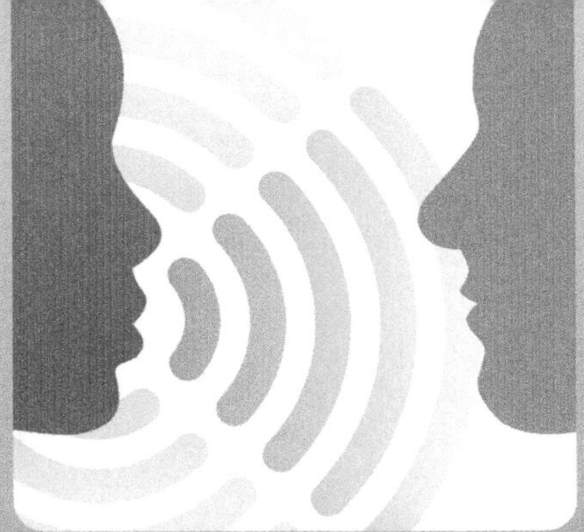

Chapter 7

Cultural pitfalls, advice on working in the UK, and culture and stress in nursing

Learning outcomes

At the end of this chapter, you should be able to:

- ✔ **identify cultural pitfalls in nursing communication**
- ✔ **consider the problems associated with moving to the UK to work or be educated in nursing**
- ✔ **identify some of the cultural issues concerned with stress in nursing**
- ✔ **consolidate some of your knowledge about culture and communication.**

Introduction

This chapter offers three things. First, it offers some examples of the cultural pitfalls that nurses in the UK can encounter. Second, it offers advice to those who are from countries other than the UK and are working here (this section, as we shall see, can also be used by students who work in nursing situations abroad). Third, it offers a case study from Brunei, conducted by the first author (PB), in which students were asked about the causes of stress in their nursing work. Therefore, this chapter summarises some of the many cultural issues that have already been discussed in this book.

Men and women

In the UK, for many decades the reality of men and women being equal has been discussed and, in many cases, practised in work and home settings, but it is not true to say that this equality has been entirely achieved. There is still an acknowledgement, for example, of the **glass ceiling**, a shorthand for the fact that women often still have more difficulty in being appointed to very senior positions than men. However, in many respects men and women are treated equally, and British people find it difficult to see why this is not a universal practice.

The truth, however, is that it is not a universal fact of life. In many countries and cultures men are seen as the decision makers, and in many ways senior to women. In certain Islamic countries, women are not allowed many of the freedoms that men in those countries take for granted. Similarly, when a husband and wife talk to a foreigner, it is usually the man who will do the talking, and who will talk on behalf of his wife. In some Islamic countries, public places are only for men, and women are not allowed to go out in the street. In others, women are not allowed to drive cars. In effect, it can mean that women are socially 'invisible'.

Again, mostly in Islamic countries, holding hands, kissing and any other form of public contact between the sexes is forbidden. However, it is not uncommon to see young men holding each other's hands, just as girls link each other's arms in the west. This is not a sign that the men are gay, but simply a sign of friendship. Similarly, in many countries, kissing on the cheek (and in some cases on the lips) is not unusual as a greeting by same-sex friends.

In nursing it is important to appreciate this different approach to the sexes. It is not sufficient to try to equalise the situation by including the woman in a conversation: it will be difficult to engage her if her husband is present. This is particularly true when the nurse is male.

Much as many of us might like to think that others *should* think about the world as we do, they do not. It would probably seem to most British people that a great injustice is being done when women are not treated as equal to men. However, it is impossible to right all the wrongs of the world, and the nurse is rarely in a position to exercise sufficient power to equalise gender relationships, and nor should they. This is not a defeatist point of view, but a realistic one. As we have already discussed, people see the world differently and behave accordingly. Although we may not agree with other people's cultural views, beliefs or practices, as nurses we should at least try to respect them (Papadopoulos, 2006).

Question for reflection

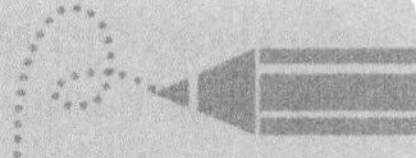

What do you feel about the nurse's role in attempting to equalise differences between attitudes towards women in different cultural groups? For example, do you believe that community nurses have a right to fight for equality for women in the community, in UK society?

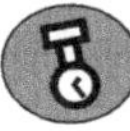

Cultural pitfalls

The UK is increasingly becoming a multicultural, multifaith society. Consequently, social, cultural and religious issues can, and often do, present a multitude of potential problems for nursing and the NHS in the UK (Papadopoulos, 2006). As discussed earlier, whereas many customs and traditions often have little or no bearing on health and health care, some social, religious and cultural beliefs can have a profound effect on a person's outlook on health, disease, illness and medical treatment. In some instances culture cannot only affect a person's understanding of illness but even their understanding of the causes of ill health (Helman, 2001). Belief and trust in a conventional medical diagnosis can also vary according to a person's social and cultural background (Andrews and Boyle, 2007).

These issues, therefore, can help to demonstrate how culture can affect a person's perspective of sickness and healing. Therefore, from a health-care perspective, understanding the patient's point of view is essential to understanding the acceptability of treatment, because if health-care provision is not seen as relevant, it may not be used or accepted by the patient (Helman, 2001). However, unfortunately, many health professionals in the UK pay very little attention, if any, to the social and cultural aspects of health and illness, which may have a direct impact on treatment and care.

Consequently, in many UK hospitals, patients with non-conventional social and cultural perspectives are often treated by health professionals with indifference, and many are even exposed to neglect, prejudice and hostility (Papadopoulos *et al*., 1994). In its worst form, this can manifest itself as racism, both personal and institutional. Factors such as language barriers and cultural differences in, for example, pain responses and sick role behaviours, may occasionally lead to some patients from minority groups being regarded as troublesome or unpopular by nurses. Social and cultural differences can also result in some patients' problems being trivialised or their seriousness not being acknowledged, whereas in other cases misdiagnosis occurs (Helman, 2001, Andrews and Boyle, 2007).

Many health professionals in the UK regard certain cultural beliefs as antiquated, illogical and even naïve, especially if physiological evidence is lacking. However, it is hoped that this book has helped to demonstrate that social and cultural beliefs are important in health care. Failure to appreciate their significance probably demonstrates a combination of ignorance and arrogance (Gill, 2000), and can cause a variety of other problems. For example, failure to understand or appreciate other people's beliefs can lead to health professionals imposing their own beliefs and values on others. Often, nurses pay little or no attention to cultural issues. However, some nurses, especially in city centre hospitals, have made an effort to acknowledge and respect patients' cultural beliefs, but although this is laudable, many such efforts have been cursory at best. A common practice in busy wards has been to compile information guidelines on common cultural and religious beliefs. Such information, however, has often been used - perhaps unthinkingly - as a mere checklist of the customs or dietary habits of certain religions or minority cultures (Mulhall, 1994). By their very nature, such guidelines also usually present a static picture of other cultures and do not allow for variations, which are common in nearly all cultures (Andrews and Boyle, 2007).

The hidden danger of such checklists is that they often lead to generalisations, causing **stereotyping**, cultural misunderstandings, prejudices and even **discrimination** (Helman, 2001). For example, labelling of patients is common: Muslims do this, Jews do that, and so on. Cultural guidelines may also discourage nurses from actively interacting with patients and their families in order to better understand their cultural beliefs and values.

Case Study

Communication about sex among British-Chinese families

Sex and sexuality is an important topic in nursing, but often difficult to talk about. In this case study, I describe some research, I, as a nurse, did into the topic of communication about sex in a particular cultural setting.

The 247 403 Chinese people living in the UK represent 0.4% of the population. This is a small, vibrant, but neglected and the least understood British minority. I was born in China and had worked there in various health-care settings before I came to the UK for further education. At the initial stage of my doctoral research, I was interested in teenage pregnancy in the UK. However, the limited research on sex-related topics among British-Chinese young people drew my attention to the study of social and cultural influences on the attitudes towards teenage sexual behaviour held by this neglected group. One of the aspects was to examine family communication about sex-related topics.

Sex is still considered a taboo subject in Chinese culture and is not discussed openly by most Chinese families, both in China and overseas. This was the case in the families I studied. Traditional attitudes to sex were most commonly held, and sexual intercourse before marriage was thought unacceptable according to Chinese cultural, philosophical and religious traditions. The families experienced a number of barriers to communication about sex. The teenagers saw the parents' limited available time as a major problem. There was also a lack of a common language between the generations, as teenagers found that they did not have the relevant Chinese vocabulary needed to discuss sex-related topics with their parents. Further barriers included embarrassment and the limited sexual knowledge and communication skills of parents. Growing up in different mainstream cultures and diverse sexual values between generations also influenced such communication. The teenagers could tell their parents everything, but not about sex, and girls thought that their parents would 'chop them to pieces' if they knew they had become sexually active.

However, they felt more comfortable talking about sex with their friends, and shared their worries and relationship problems with them. Although such communication was limited in these families, parents tended to convey their sexual values using various strategies, including speaking Chinese at home, commenting on television programmes, and supervising outings and friendships.

A number of recommendations can be put forward as to how nurses who are involved in the provision of sexual health services could be made to work differently and more effectively. Some of the difficulties faced by British-Chinese families have been found in the wider population; however, nurses need to be aware of specific barriers these families may encounter, including parents' lack

of time and language issues. They can stress the moral aspects of sex more, promote parents' communication skills, and help them overcome barriers by providing a resource list of relevant material, literature and websites. There is also the need to actively respect the views of minority ethnic people, and to tailor sexual health services to the needs of young people from culturally diverse backgrounds.

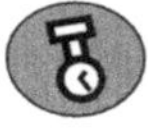

Advice on working in the UK or in other countries

Although this section is written from the perspective of a nurse coming to work in the UK, it can also be used as a selection of issues to be thought about by a UK student or qualified nurse going to work in another country.

Working in another country can be both eye opening and a source of 'culture shock'. Culture shock is the feeling we get when all our usual norms and values are suddenly overturned (Barnard and Spencer, 2002). Some cultures, for example, predominantly use spoons to eat with, and rarely or never use a fork. However, in the UK, people usually eat with a knife and fork and put the fork in their mouths. Similarly, in some cultures (as discussed earlier), students listen carefully to their teachers, are polite to them, and rarely ask questions of them. In the UK, students seem not only to interrupt teachers and challenge them, but are encouraged to do so.

In clinical practice, nurses in the UK may have a much more casual relationship with doctors than is the case in many other countries. As these differences in values and practice add up, so can the sense of alienation and of culture shock. This can often lead to those new to the UK wanting to go home, to seek out friends from their own background, wanting things to be 'different' and more 'normal', and so on. Therefore, in this chapter we offer some tips for coping with the stress that can arise out of working in the UK, particularly if you have previously worked in a very different culture.

It should be noted that people vary immensely in their ability to adapt to different circumstances. There is no 'normal' way of reacting to change of this sort. Some people find a two-week holiday in another country stressful, whereas others gladly do voluntary work in an entirely different culture, for months or years, and find the whole process relatively unstressful. Allow - and perhaps even expect - yourself to be stressed at first, but remember that you are not the first, nor the last, person to have moved to the UK from another country and made a success of it.

Preparation

First, you must prepare for working in the UK. Above all, make sure your paperwork, visas and preparation for registration as a nurse are all in order. When these things go wrong, it can be particularly worrying and only adds to the level of cultural strangeness that can be felt. Generally speaking, the agencies that deal with visas and work permits in the UK are not as bureaucratic or officious as they can be in other countries. However, they still require certain standards to be met, and that papers are in order. Get all this sorted out well in advance. Your local school of nursing may be able to help you, or advise you of who to contact for further help, support or advice.

Work on your language

If your first language is not English, then try to make sure that you have had sufficient lessons in that language before you arrive in the UK. Remember, though, that just as is the case in your own country, accents vary considerably, even in a small set of countries such as the UK. You will probably have been taught to speak English with a particular accent (probably English or North American). English spoken in England, Wales, Scotland and Northern Ireland may sound very different to the type of English you have been taught or have listened to at home. Wherever possible, in the UK, speak English and try to resist the temptation to slip back into your own language at the first opportunity. Students' English can improve dramatically in about 2 months if they really concentrate on speaking the language most of the time.

Try to make a range of friends

It is always tempting to seek out friends from our own country or culture. This is normal. If you really want to learn more about the English language and UK culture, try to make friends from various places, and particularly British friends. This will help you to understand those aspects of the language that are most difficult to acquire: idiom and humour. In any language, 'short' phrases often replace the more technically correct ones and it is important to try to absorb these idiomatic expressions early on, for patients as well as staff will often use them.

If you are able to make new friends, go to different sorts of social events and try different foods. You may not like them at first, but you may well be surprised at what you find yourself eating. Clearly you need also to observe the rules about eating laid down by your own particular religion or culture. Note that religion may well not play such a large part in society in the UK as it does in your own country. Try not to be surprised that many people in the UK will not talk about religion, and many will claim not to have a religion. If you have very strong religious beliefs yourself, maintain them while you work in the UK (provided of course you want to) and do try not to let them slip. If you do, you may find it very difficult to fit back into the country you return to. Working in another country is often a balance between holding on to one's own culture and absorbing parts of another.

Be observant

Start off from the point of view that things will be different in the UK and that people will act differently. Quietly observe the ways in which nurses, doctors and patients talk to each other and act towards one another. At first you may not particularly agree with the way things are done, but, like anyone learning about another country's cultural traditions, beliefs and way of life, this is the fact of culture in the UK. Slowly try to model yourself on some of the better practice that you see. Again, this does not mean throwing off your own cultural values and practices (you probably cannot do this anyway), but it does mean that you will increasingly develop confidence in your own practice. If you are attending study days in a school of nursing, try to pluck up the courage to raise questions, or even to disagree with what the lecturer is saying. You will find UK nurse teachers generally easy to talk to and to discuss things with.

Use this book 'backwards'

This book has been about how to help UK nurses to become more culturally aware. You can use it to see the sorts of issue that UK students need to think about when trying to understand other cultures, so in this sense you can use the book in reverse. Use it to identify the anxieties that UK students and nurses may have when faced with cultural issues different from their own. You may be surprised at how similar those anxieties are to your own. Further, you can, of course, help to raise awareness of relevant social, cultural and religious issues at a local level, by informing the nurses and other health professionals that you work with about your own culture.

Studying in the UK

Teaching and learning methods used in the UK may be different from those you are used to in your home country. As we have noted, in the west generally there has been a move over the past 40 years towards 'student-centred learning', in which the student plays just as important a part in his or her learning as does the teacher. In this approach, the student no longer passively accepts knowledge from a higher authority - the teacher - but is prepared to learn how to find out information for him or herself, and also to debate, in a critical way, the knowledge that is discussed with the teacher. All of this takes some getting used to if you have come from a culture where the teacher is very much the authority and 'in charge'. At first, you may be upset and even insulted by the teacher's apparently casual manner, and by the fact that a fairly equal relationship can exist between teachers and students.

The main teaching methods used in the UK and the west are the **lecture**, the **seminar**, the **tutorial** and various workshop techniques.

The lecture

This form of teaching is well known around the world. Typically, a lecture lasts between 40 and 90 minutes, during which the lecturer does most of the talking, usually highlighting the talk with a PowerPoint (a Microsoft presentation software program) presentation. Following (and often during, if the session is interactive) the lecture there may or may not be a period for questions and, in the UK, if a question period is allowed, students will generally ask questions freely and be prepared to challenge the lecturer on what he or she has said. In the UK this is not seen as rudeness or lack of respect, but as part of the learning experience.

The seminar

The typical seminar focuses on one or a small group of students who prepare a 'paper' that forms the basis of a discussion. In some seminars, the student or students begin by reading the paper through, although use is increasingly being made of PowerPoint for a short presentation on the material. The topic of the seminar may be set by the teacher, or may be chosen by the student or students. Following the short presentation, all of the other students and the teacher will engage in a detailed discussion of what has been talked about to that point. The teacher will not necessarily take the lead in this discussion, and indeed may take a fairly low-key part. Nor is it considered necessary for the teacher to have the final word on the topic, or to 'correct' the students.

The tutorial

Tutorials are one-to-one sessions with a teacher. Normally, prior to the meeting the student will have sent a hard copy of what they are working on, or an e-mail copy of it, to the teacher, who will have read the work before the two parties meet. The tutorial offers both the student and the teacher time to discuss issues, and the student is expected to be able to defend his or her work. Again, the student does not go to the tutorial simply to learn from the teacher: both parties can learn from this method.

Workshop approaches

Workshops can range from half a day to a week in duration. Usually they involve some short lectures, a great deal of discussion and some experiential learning activities, such as role-play and simulation or, perhaps, discussion in pairs. The aim of a workshop is normally to pool learning resources (from both staff and students) so that both may learn. Again, do not expect that the workshop leader (often known as a facilitator) will automatically 'take charge'. Often, on a more than one-day workshop the first session is for participants to decide on the content and structure of the workshop. The facilitator, in this case, does not impose his or her own structure on the workshop but allows that structure to grow out of this initial discussion.

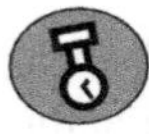

General points about teaching and learning in the UK

Both male and female teachers and lecturers are equally respected in the UK. Titles such as 'Doctor' and 'Professor' are used more rarely when addressing a teacher, and many teachers prefer to be called by their first names. Students from some cultures find this situation difficult or even impossible, and continue to use the more formal form of address. Do not worry if this applies to you, as lecturers will have come across this situation before. Do try, however, to join in the spirit of student-centred learning. Even if it is at first very difficult to believe that a teacher is not setting him or herself up in authority, it can soon become apparent that both students and teachers have much to learn from one another.

Assessment of student work in the UK often takes the form of written assignments or essays. You may or may not be used to this approach, and if you have lived in a country where assessment of what you have learnt is often carried out through set questions and examination, writing assignments can initially be daunting. Structuring your work can help. Be clear about the aim of your assignment, and define the terms that you are using. Go to the internet and the library to identify what has been written on this topic before (and particularly what research has been done on the topic) and then, slowly, learn to summarise it. Later on, it is to be hoped that you will also be able to be critical of the theory and research that you have read. Your assignment will then contain a discussion of what you have read and reach a conclusion. It may close with suggestions for further work that needs to be done in the field. Once again, this sort of work relies on *you* looking for information and not just relying on the teacher to give you that information. Most teachers and lecturers will, of course, be prepared to help you, and you are likely to be given a personal tutor to help you work through your early assignments.

Teaching and learning in the UK can be a very different experience from the educational activities found in some other countries. Part of learning about the culture of a country includes learning about the way in which people in that country learn themselves. Try to remain open minded, try to join in the discussions, and try to appreciate what is at the heart of the student-centred approach: it is a method that helps people to become lifelong learners. Few of us, once we leave school, colleges or universities, regularly get 'taught' again, but rely on the skills we have learned to teach ourselves. For example, we are both university academics (PB is a university professor and PG is a university senior research fellow) and so do not often go on formal learning courses in the same way as an undergraduate or newly qualified nurse might. However, because we have both grown up with the student-centred approach to learning, we can readily find out what we need to know from the internet, libraries, and discussing things with other people. We may not keep huge amounts of information in our heads, but we know where to find it when we need to.

In the final section of this chapter, a case study on stress and nursing among students in Brunei is discussed. The aim of this is to highlight some of the many cultural issues that have already been discussed in this book. It is also notable that in an international study of stress in student nurses in Albania, Brunei, the Czech Republic, Malta and Wales (Burnard *et al.*, 2008) it was found that stress was reported as highest in Bruneian students. A considerable amount of this stress might be accountable for in terms of cultural influences. As you read this, try to compare the Bruneian experience of being a nurse with your own.

Case Study

Stress in Bruneian students

This section offers the direct thoughts of a group of 20 student nurses from Brunei about what stressed them in their nurse training. It is included here to illustrate the way some of the principles in this book 'come alive' in the real nursing situation. It therefore helps to demonstrate culture at work in nursing.

The 20 students were interviewed individually, and then the data from those interviews were analysed using a process of thematic content analysis (Burnard, 1991). The findings from the study were organised under the three headings identified by Carson and Kuipers (1998) in a previous, related study: stressors; things that moderate stress; and the outcomes of being stressed. Where appropriate, verbatim quotes from participants have also been included to help demonstrate key findings.

Brunei is a small, oil-rich Islamic state in northwest Borneo. It has a total land area of 5765 km^2, with a coastline facing the South China Sea, and a population of about 357 800. It shares a common border with the Malaysian state of Sarawak. In cultural terms, Brunei is a collectivist (as opposed to an individualist) culture, with a strong emphasis on the centrality of the family and on the 'group' rather than on the 'individual', as noted in earlier chapters.

Question for reflection

As you read these accounts of Bruneian students' views of stress in nursing, compare and contrast them to your own views. In what way does nursing in Brunei seem similar to nursing in the UK, and in what way is it different? If you come from outside the UK, to what degree are these accounts similar (or dissimilar) to your own feelings about stress in nursing?

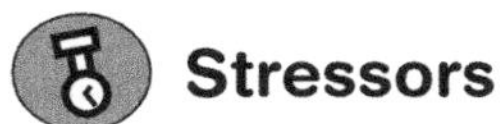

Stressors

Nursing as a stressful activity

A number of Bruneian students were able to define, in general terms, what they meant by the term 'stress' and how both clinical and academic aspects of nursing contributed to it:

Stress is very common in nursing. My definition is that it is a mental disorder because it affects our mental state and involves us emotionally. As a student, I have been going to clinical placement and I have found stress in the hospital. Some of the pressure is peer pressure and sometimes it is from other staff and lack of facilities in the hospital - sometimes poor management. At the end of the day I feel very stressed.

When we talk about nursing in Brunei, the facilities for students are limited - the library is short of books and papers. Organisation of time is another factor, but facilities are the most stressful thing.

Well, what is stressful in nursing is the way it is managed. The system, the nursing schedule, sometimes the people and the environment, both in the college and in the clinical setting, are stressful.

These responses point to the emotional aspects of stress and some of the broad causes of that emotional response, in both clinical and academic settings, with emphasis placed on both people and environmental considerations, themes that were developed in more detail in these and other interviews.

Clinical stressors: 'wearing pink'

The wearing of a pink uniform denotes the grade of a student nurse and seems to symbolise that status for a number of Bruneian students. Indeed, the wearing of the pink uniform appears to inform other staff of how they might react to the students. Brunei is a hierarchical society, and in the nursing profession it would appear that those who wear pink may occupy the lower rungs of that hierarchy. This, in turn, causes stress for some students.

We are wearing a pink uniform and the staff nurses wear a different colour, and this creates a barrier and we cannot object to anything when we are criticised; we can't answer back. This can be stressful.

Because we are still students and attached to clinical areas, sometimes we have to adapt very quickly to the environment, get to know the other staff, the doctors (what they like and what they don't like) and most of our opinions may not be acceptable. We are still students, so we cannot say very much - we are wearing the pink uniform.

The question of status in the nursing hierarchy was a theme for many of the Bruneian students. They often felt that being students, in the clinical setting, meant that they experience a sense of tension. On the one hand, their lowly status may make it difficult to receive help from others, and on the other hand senior staff may expect them to have certain knowledge and skills that they felt they did not possess. However, the degree to which this was stressful varied:

It is the staff there [in the clinical setting]. Because sometimes I don't feel very good in doing the skills and I feel they criticise me. Clinical practice isn't always stressful: sometimes it is.

Lack of communication between the staff, in the clinical setting is very stressful - there is a distance between students and trained staff.

Sometimes, too, the volume of work expected of students was seen as a stressor, and in some cases the uncertainty of what might be expected led students to doubt their own ability:

In clinical it is stressful because of workload, and sometimes the nurses tend to ask students to do all the simple things, like taking temperatures, taking patients to X-ray and so on – they are more likely to ask students to do that; we have to do so much.

I like the clinical work but I find it very stressful, and more stressful than working in the college. We are new and we do not have much experience, and this gives me a very stressful feeling when I do not have the skills I feel I should have.

A constant theme throughout the study was the relationships between the students and the trained staff. If the trained staff were prepared to help the students, support and teach them, stress seemed less evident. However, often it appeared that senior staff would not adopt this teaching and supporting role, but expected students to still be able to demonstrate nursing skills and knowledge:

Somehow, in the clinical area, if we are very close to one person, they tend to show you how that area works, but if you do not get close to a person, you may be just told to get on with it . . . If communication is not very good, in the clinical setting, sometimes staff talk about you behind your back.

There is only one thing that is stressful in clinical practice and that is mingling with the seniors, who look down on us and who do not want to teach us.

From my point of view, when it comes to working in the ward with the senior staff, there is not very good communication – we are new in the wards and not superior – that is stressful.

It sometimes appeared to be a case of the degree to which students could 'manage' other people. One student suggested the difference between the clinical setting and the academic setting in terms of this type of management:

It is more stressful in the clinical area because in the college* we can deal with the teachers *and they know how we feel. [emphasis added]

Caring for patients was also another source of stress. The human element of nursing and the fact of caring for a range of physical, psychological and social issues meant for many students that nursing was more stressful than other occupations. Sometimes this stress was also linked to staff shortages:

For me, nursing is more stressful than other jobs because we are dealing with human beings, not only to cure them, but we deal with their physical, psychological and psychosocial [problems].

We care about people's lives, so it is more stressful. Teachers, for example, just give knowledge, but we care about people, so I think it is much more stressful. There are a lot of tasks to do with people in nursing.

Nursing is stressful, it is a very stressful job because when I did my occupational health option, I visited a website and it showed nursing to be one of the most stressful occupations. I think it is, because in clinical nursing we have to care for people in a ward, and there are too many patients and too big a workload. There is conflict with colleagues, doctors, relatives, and even the patients themselves.

Academic stress and 'paperwork'

College life and the nursing education system were other sources of stress for some Bruneian students. Various themes were frequently mentioned: having to complete assignments and dissertations, the organisation and changing nature of the college, and the college environment itself. Often, the written work was referred to as 'paperwork', perhaps to be contrasted with the more practical or hands-on approach taken in the clinical setting.

I guess working in the college is more stressful than clinical – you tend to have to do more paperwork. It is the time management that is difficult.

It is more stressful in the college because I love to work in the clinical area. When I am in the college I have to think about my paperwork, the dissertation, the exams, the people around me, the study schedule, and then we have to wait for an hour to have a good class, we have to transfer from one class to another. The college sometimes does not have a proper system for managing learning. I have to travel a long way, too.

For some, the written work at college was extremely stressful. The following respondent enumerated some of the things that she found stressful about college work, and notes that the dissertation, in particular, was the most stressful activity she had taken part in to date:

In the college we are stressed because we have to learn a lot of theory, and every year we have our assignments to do and these are very stressful. We didn't have much guidance for the dissertations. The dissertation was the most stressful thing I have done in my life. Sometimes we have to do lectures in front of peers, and that is very stressful, particularly when the lecturer gives you the title very late.

Language

In Brunei, nursing is taught in English but practised in Malay. This was a source of stress for some of the students.

We have presentations in front of our colleagues, our English is not good, and we tend to feel down and have negative thinking. I feel my English is not good, due to teachers I

cannot understand, and explain: they cannot understand, and it causes us to fail English tests.

In the college, studying in English is the main problem for most of the students in Brunei. I like to learn in English, but I have difficulty in understanding sometimes; that's why I feel stressed.

Discussions with the educational staff of the college also identified the fact that those students who can write better English than others tend to be more successful in their examinations and to have higher marks in their assignments and dissertations.

Diplomas and degrees

Another source of stress, not directly related to the experience of working in the clinical setting or in the college, was concern about whether or not a diploma programme was sufficient as a primary nursing qualification. There was discussion about the fact that, in other countries, it was possible to study for a Bachelor's degree in the same time that Bruneian students study for a diploma in nursing:

In Brunei we still only have a diploma course, and I feel we should have a degree course. In other countries, they take the same time to do a degree as we do to do a diploma. We do not want to be left behind.

For me, in Brunei, just to get the diploma in this country takes longer than it does in other countries. In Singapore, for example, you can get a degree in the same time as it takes to get a diploma here.

At the time of writing, a degree course curriculum has been developed in Brunei and it is hoped to offer an initial degree in nursing very soon.

Dislocation: between two lives

The result of learning the 'ideal' in school and facing the 'reality' of the clinical setting sometimes caused tension in the students. This tension was also compounded by the problem of attempting to divide time between working in the clinical setting and completing assignments and the dissertation. Thus we noted a sense of dislocation: a sense of being divided between both the 'lives' of the college and of the clinic and the 'lives' as illustrated by two different languages. For translation between two languages is always a matter of negotiation: it cannot be assumed that the concepts and ideas of one language can always be perfectly translated into another. The students in this study had to make that 'translation' themselves. They were required to learn in English and then translate the theories and concepts they learned into clinical practice in Malay.

In all of this was the need to learn nursing 'properly' and how to nurse in an appropriate and sensitive manner. Sometimes, students appreciated that what they saw qualified nurses (and sometimes doctors) doing was not how they wanted to nurse themselves. Sometimes they silently questioned whether or not what they were being taught and what they observed in clinical practice was conducive to good nursing care.

The following student summarised some of these tensions, between what he felt was 'good nursing' and good clinical supervision and what he saw in practice, as follows:

As a student most of the stress comes from clinical areas. When there is a problem between student and mentor, in the the way of supervision, the supervisor may 'let go' of the student. Sometimes the supervisor gives autonomy, for the tasks that have to be done, to the student, but sometimes overlooks that supervision is needed. The stress is because of the way the task might affect the patient. Then we have to try to get supervision from other staff nurses. But we cannot question the credibility of the staff nurses because they do not stick to procedures such as handwashing, e.g. a staff nurse in supervision said that handwashing is waste of time, due to pressure of time. A student is stressed because he does not want to be like that: a staff nurse is adopting this behaviour and it is worrying. Stress is due to patients not being cared for the way they should be . . . I have even

seen some doctors insult patients. Fussy patients are talked about by the staff nurses, and it upsets me to see this. I would rather die straightaway than be nursed by those nurses. I don't want to die a slow and grim death.

Being stressed

Students described what it was like to experience stress. Sometimes, stress produced somatic symptoms as well as psychological ones, and sometimes it changed appetites:

I feel a headache and sometimes – not really a mental block, but I cannot do things when I am stressed; it distracts me and stops me from doing things. It makes me a little upset, but I do not cry.

I get a migraine; I just want to bang my head against the wall and shout.

It's kind of like rough: I feel like shouting and I become angry, even towards the person closest to me. In my stressed mood I get a high-pitched voice.

When I am stressed I eat a lot. Stress really, really affects my mood and my relationships with friends.

For me, when I am stressed, I feel like eating too much. It has a negative impact and a positive one. In a positive way I learn how to improve myself and how to cope with work; in a negative way I like to eat more, and this is not good. Also, stress is not good for mental health.

I don't know how to deal with the stress. Sometimes I don't eat.

Often, psychological symptoms of stress were described by the students: feelings of depression, anger, tension and anxiety. At times of stress, as we shall see, some wanted to be with friends but others wanted to hide themselves away until the stress feelings had passed. Examples of the students' views about their psychological stress symptoms were:

Well, I feel long and short term my mood and behaviour changing, negative thinking; long term I feel just lonely, don't want to speak to anyone - my self-esteem is low, confidence low.

I just keep myself in the room and rest: I do not want to think any more until the stress has gone. I also lose my temper sometimes. I don't want to talk to anyone.

I feel I can't really do anything. I feel like crying, and normally I would look for my friends to have a laugh or something. I try not to be angry with people but sometimes I am without realising it.

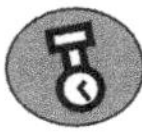

Moderators

Moderators are the processes that are used to either relieve stress or modify it into a form that makes it acceptable. Students used a range of moderating processes to relieve their stress.

Interpersonal issues

Stress was often moderated through other people. Students spoke to friends, to their tutors, and sometimes - but by no means always - to their parents. Some felt that talking about stress, or factors that caused stress, with their families simply burdened them.

I talk with my friends, sometimes they joke with me; they take me window shopping, or we go to the cinema, and also I call my parents.

I watch TV or go out with friends. Also we eat. I can talk to my friends about things that stress me, but if they are

personal I keep them to myself. I can also talk to my sisters - one of my sisters is also a nurse. I can talk to my mum, but mostly I keep things from her.

The social and 'joking' function of friends was often referred to: it would appear that rather than having 'deep' discussions about stress, the function of friends was often to joke and help relieve the tension. Sometimes, friends were chatted to after the initial feelings of stress had passed. In the following example, the student does not appear to need friends while acutely stressed, and prefers not to worry her parents about her stress:

I don't talk to my friends until I have calmed down - after a few days. I do need friends to talk to, but not immediately when I feel stressed. I do not share with my parents when I am stressed - I do not want to make them more stressed about my studies because they are paying for my studies - I do not want to make them feel anxious.

Similarly, another student preferred to attempt to calm herself first, before talking to friends. If this failed, friends or tutors could help:

If I am stressed I feel I don't want to talk to anyone: I want to think about my problem on my own. If I cannot, I will find someone I really trust and who can help me, like my husband. If he cannot help, I can talk to a best friend or a tutor.

Trusted friends

A number of the Bruneian students said that they could talk about their stress to 'trusted friends'. These trusted friends could be described and compared and contrasted with more general friends, or 'friends you hang out with'.

Trusted friends are ones who understand me at the same level, depth. Trusted friends are ones you can share your

feelings with, but not, normally, your depression. Trusted friends are normally my age.

A trusted friend is someone you can trust, someone you are really close to, someone who knows your background, someone who understands your feelings and who is much the same as myself. Other sorts of friends are just ones you hang out with.

For one respondent, the issue of having trusted friends was a vital one. Other sorts of friends might not be reliable, or they might even be potentially threatening:

It is not easy to find a trusted friend, some friends are back-stabbers. When you face difficulties they just drift away from you and back-stab. A trusted friend will help you in difficulties and help you out. Sometimes there is bullying: I was bullied. I nearly quit: they were not good. 'Trusted friend': someone you can confide in. Other friends are just ones to hang out with and have fun with.

However, as noted above, just having friends to 'hang out with' was sometimes important as a means of reducing stress levels:

I like to make jokes, cheer up the day, mingle around with friends, also do something like listening to music, surfing the internet. Hang out with friends.

Sports and hobbies

A number of students referred to sports and other hobbies as means of moderating or relieving stress. Sporting activities were sometimes arranged by the nursing college, but some students chose to take part in sporting activities independently:

I also play sports, so I think that I give out all of my stress in my sports – I play netball and badminton – this is organised by the college.

I prefer to go bowling and do some outdoor activities - go to the beach. I talk to my friends: they are very supportive, and my family are also supportive.

Sometimes I will go swimming, jogging, hiking.

Prayer and nature

For some, a form of communion with nature was a means of reducing or relieving stress. This was sometimes linked to a religious theme:

Above all, I go to lonely places, lakes, appreciate God's creation.

When I am stressed I go to the sea and shout at the sea.

The latter response seemed to be a form of both catharsis and social isolation: it seemed important to be able to get away from others, but also to have some form of 'safe' emotional release.

Other ways of coping with stress

Individual students identified particular, sometimes idiosyncratic, ways of dealing with stress. One, for example, suggested:

Sometimes when I get home from work I like to put the music on very loud and drive so fast.

Another student identified a range of strategies that she used to moderate the effects of work- and study-related stress:

We have counsellors who can help, in the hospital, for all the working people, if they have stress. Some people feel guilty about seeing a counsellor and say 'talk to your friends and family'. I like to talk to my mother, my family and my friends and share with them what makes me feel stressed and seek their help. With humour I deal with it also, and I also like to relax by listening to music, doing tai chi. Sometimes if I cannot cope, I cry and this helps to release tensions.

This student notes the availability of a counsellor to help 'all the working people', but also alludes to a certain stigma attached to going to see such a person. In collectivist cultures, it is frequently the case that people will talk about their problems most readily to their family and friends, rather than to a disinterested outsider. This student also summarises a range of methods discussed by many of her colleagues in the study: crying, using humour, relaxing by listening to music, and talking to friends and family.

Organisational and institutional moderators

Many students could articulate what they felt could be done, within the nursing profession, to lessen stress. These ideas might be thought of as 'organisational moderators'. Examples included the following. In the first, the student felt that 'someone' should be made responsible for the issue of stress, and also noted staff and equipment shortages:

Nursing should provide a consultant who can solve the problem. Also, I think that nursing officers should be able to work alongside doctors without bias. The stressed person should be able to talk to someone who they can trust. Shortage of staff is also a cause of stress, and the lack of appropriate equipment - sometimes we only have one thermometer, for example.

Another student identified the human and caring features that needed to be attended to in order to reduce stress, perhaps thereby identifying a 'core' aspect of the health-care professions-patient relationship:

It goes back to patient care: doctors need to respect patients, and give a feeling of really caring, as well as nurses, for the patient and family. Not all do at the moment. New doctors are better and there are signs of change. Latest things on internet, research on patient-centred bedside care - this will help all.

Finally, in this short selection, a student suggested that nursing should be acknowledged as a stressful occupation and that organisational arrangements should be made to help people to cope with it:

One thing we can start with is student life itself: providing good facilities and preparing them with ways to cope with stress. It is never openly said that nursing is stressful, and I would appreciate it if they could give us some hints about how to cope - it is a bit pressurised in the college. And also the environment of the college needs to be considered - some places to relax and chill out.

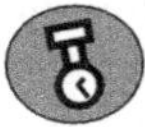

Outcomes

The use of moderators of stress seemed in most cases to relieve that stress, if only temporarily. A number of students also noted that there were both positive and negative effects of stress, particularly *unmoderated* stress.

Positive outcomes: being motivated

For some students stress could be a motivator: it could force them to reconsider his or her position and challenge them to do something:

Yes, I guess. Everyone has stress. Everyone has to deal with it. Sometimes stress can make us self-motivated. It makes you think further and further.

We can learn to cope with it; we learn how to cope with difficult situations.

One good effect is that it changes us to make us manage ourselves properly.

I think, in a way, it is important for one to have stress: it is a signal to say 'Hello. This is too much.' This is one of the best things about stress. With proper management, it

is healthy to have some stress. Everyone has stress. Even if your pockets are filled with money, you still have stress.

The last student, quoted above, notes both the 'warning call' of stress and also a way of rationalising stress by appreciating that 'everyone has stress'. However, one student felt unable to find anything positive in stress and suggested:

I don't think there are good effects of stress.

Negative outcomes: depression and mental illness

Negative effects, particularly long-term effects, were also noted by the students. They included the idea that stress could cause depression and other mental illness. Long-term stress might also cause students to leave their training. However, one student seemed particularly aware of the immediate as well as the long-term effects. She noted not only that stress might lead to mental illness, but that you might lose friends in the process:

I find stress is always negative, and it can give you mental problems and you will be like in stress all of the time and ignored by people and you let it out to people and you will lose people – they will just go. If you are not stressed, people will come to you. If you are stressed, people will leave you.

For others, negative views of stress were almost the mirror image of positive ones: stress could be demotivating:

I think stress can demotivate you. You feel uncomfortable and do not accept what people say to you, and you feel unlikeable. You work with less confidence and you feel lost in the ward. You become lonely and don't want to talk to people, and you say to yourself: 'I am not that good'.

Again, the suggestion is that stress can make you unpopular. This may go some way to explaining some students' reluctance to talk to friends and family about stress. Again, in collectivist cultures, a sense of inclusion and a sense of oneness with friends and family is very important.

Ideal type

An 'ideal type' is an idealised world picture of a person, emerging from the data. This was originally described by Max Weber (Coser, 1977). The following is the ideal type that emerges from the data in this study, that is, a summary of the key features of a Bruneian nursing student. It should be useful, in the future, to compare and contrast this with other ideal types emerging from other cultural studies of stress of the same sort. The ideal type is as follows:

The Bruneian nursing student comes from a close family background. She is usually Muslim. She has a circle of friends, some of whom are trusted friends: people she can talk to about problems, and to whom she will turn before she talks to her parents. Others are simply friends to have fun with - and 'having fun' or joking is an important feature of friendship. In clinical nursing, she finds herself having low status and may or may not be helped to learn by more senior staff. In the nursing college, she finds the physical environment not always conducive to study and finds learning resources sparse. She sometimes feels overwhelmed by the diet of assignments and by completing the dissertation. Having to learn and write in English, not her native language (Malay), causes problems. Out of all this she experiences stress. This manifests itself in various ways: sometimes she feels like crying, and sometimes she wants to shut herself away in her room. To alleviate the stress she may engage in sporting activities, listen to music or talk to her trusted friends. She may not immediately talk to her parents, for fear of worrying them unnecessarily. She feels that both the nursing college and the clinical

settings could be better organised and resourced, and realises that shortage of clinical staff contributes to work-related stress.

Conclusion

This chapter has explored some of the key pitfalls associated with social, cultural and religious issues that nurses can encounter in the UK and other countries. We have also offered some practical advice to nurses from other countries who may be contemplating working in the UK. And finally this chapter has presented an empirical case study from Brunei of stress in nursing. It is therefore hoped that this chapter has further demonstrated how culture and associated issues can affect nursing and nursing practice. The final chapter in this book explores cultural awareness.

Suggested reading

Helman C (2007). *Culture, Health and Illness*, 5th edn. London: Hodder Arnold.

Hobfoll SE (2004). *Stress, Culture and Community: the Psychology and Philosophy of Stress.* London: Kluwer.

Papadopoulos I (2006). *Transcultural Health and Social Care: Development of Culturally Competent Practitioners*. London: Churchill Livingstone.

Rice VH (2000). *Handbook of Stress, Coping and Health: Implications for Nursing Research, Theory and Practice*. London: Sage.

Saunders G (1994). *A History of Brunei*. Oxford: Oxford University Press.

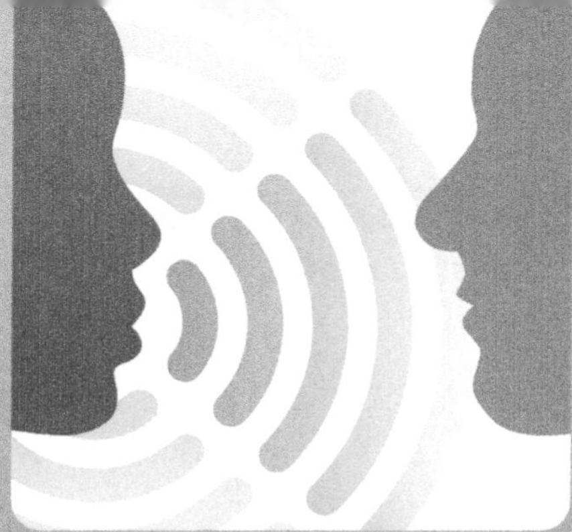

Chapter 8

Developing cultural awareness

Learning outcomes

At the end of this chapter, you should be able to:

- ✔ identify the concept of cultural awareness
- ✔ consider some of the things you might do to enhance your own cultural awareness
- ✔ discuss ways of incorporating cultural issues into your own nursing care

Introduction

Having discussed how social, cultural and religious issues can affect health and illness, this chapter concludes by exploring how we can better appreciate other people's beliefs. In order to offer the best care we can to patients from diverse cultures and subcultures, we need to develop cultural awareness. This chapter identifies some of the key elements of such awareness, and describes how it can be developed in everyday life and in nursing practice.

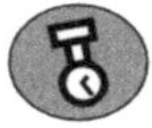

Aspects of cultural awareness

The following is a short list of elements of cultural awareness. It is not claimed to be comprehensive, but it is suggested that paying attention to these elements will help you to be more aware of how you consider and care for people from other cultures.

- Information
- Empathy
- Open-mindedness
- Interest in others
- Willingness to learn from others
- Lack of prejudice.

Information

Knowing something about the culture of a particular person or group is a good starting point for developing cultural awareness. Consider the following ideas. At the time of writing this book, and probably at the time of your reading it, there is tension between many Christian cultures and many Islamic cultures. Consider how much you know about either of these cultures. You are probably more likely to know more about Islam if you are Muslim than you are likely to know about Christianity if you are a Christian. This sounds strange, but it remains a fact that Islamic teaching is generally more thorough (and begins at a younger age) than is the case with Christianity. In the west, many people are what might be called 'nominal Christians', i.e. they claim to be Christian simply on the basis of their parents having been so, or because they are not sure about what other religious options they may have. On the other hand, a Muslim person will normally be very clear about what Islam involves and what it is to be a Muslim.

It is possible to develop knowledge about other cultures on a little-by-little basis. As you care for different people from different cultures, get in the habit of looking up information about those particular cultures. The internet is often a good place to start. Also, it is quite reasonable to ask people about their culture (Papadopoulos, 2006). In fact, provided the patient or their family are happy to discuss such issues with you, speaking to people is one of the best ways of understanding them better. Most of us are only too pleased that some other person is taking an interest in us. Remember, too, that the individual's view of a culture will often tell you a great deal about that particular person. Written material on culture tends to generalise, as discussed in the previous chapter, and not every person in a given culture is likely to perceive things in the same way (Helman, 2001). Furthermore, written material often presents a rather 'static' picture of a given culture, and usually does not allow for subtle differences or variations (Helman, 2001).

Question for reflection

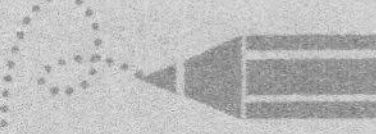

In what ways have you noticed this book generalising about culture? In what ways do you think you vary from any descriptions about your culture mentioned in this book?

Accurate information about a culture can help us to understand how the person in front of us has developed his or her own views about the world, and how his or her background and socialisation have added to those views.

Another way of attempting to understand other cultural viewpoints is to study the literature, poetry, music and art of those cultures. Often fiction and art can represent cultural points of view more powerfully than can non-fiction books and research reports. Consider, for example, how rap music, country and western, rock and roll, classical, rhythm and blues, drum and bass all convey particular subcultures, and how different they are. Note, also, your own reaction to these types of music. What are the options? You may like one or more of the categories, or you may like none. You may like another musical option, not identified in that list. Whatever sort of music you like, it is arguably conveying certain cultural and subcultural values. Similarly, novels and poetry written within a certain culture convey much about the country and culture in which they were written. Perhaps the most accessible means of doing this, from a UK point of view, is to read novels written by British and North American authors, and to listen to UK and North American music. It will soon be appreciated that although English is spoken in both countries, the two cultures are quite different. It is sometimes said of the USA and the UK that they are two countries divided by the same language. You can note, also, that even the use of English in the USA and the UK varies considerably. If this is so, imagine how different views of the world vary when different languages are involved. For language is what helps us to define the world. We understand the world through the language we use, and there is often no direct relationship between one language and another (Barnard and Spencer, 2002). This soon becomes apparent when you study a second, third or fourth language. It soon becomes clear that some cultural concepts simply cannot be conveyed in the language of another culture. Try as we might to understand other cultures, we may never do so completely.

As you will have appreciated through having read this far, the first author (PB) has spent a lot of time doing cultural research in Thailand. Consequently, I (PB) have sometimes found myself pondering on what it might be like to 'become Thai'. I do not mean this simply from the point of view of changing my nationality and by learning the language fluently, but from the view of what it might be to change one's cultural being into something else. You will probably not be surprised to appreciate that I decided it was impossible. Perhaps it is impossible ultimately to change our culture so completely that we become a member of another culture (particularly if it is profoundly different from our own), unless the move to that culture takes place at a very early age.

Empathy

Empathy is the ability to enter the perceptual world of the other person: to see the world as they see it. It also suggests an ability to convey this identification of feelings to the other person.

Empathy is clearly different from sympathy. Sympathy suggests feeling sorry for the other person, or perhaps identifying with how they feel. If I sympathise, I imagine myself being in the other person's position and imagine how I would feel. If I empathise, however, I try to imagine how it is to *be* the other person – feeling sorry for him does not really come into it.

To empathise with another person, then, is to put your own feelings, thoughts and beliefs to one side and to try to view the world from that person's perspective. None of this is easy. We seem to have an inbuilt tendency to judge what other people say as 'right' or 'wrong' according to the degree to which we do or do not agree with it. To empathise, you must really try to put yourself second and the person in front of you first. In learning to empathise and understand what it might be like to be that person is an excellent way of developing and enhancing cultural awareness. It is debatable whether you can teach someone to be truly empathetic, but nurses, because of the very nature of their profession, often find it easier to develop such skills.

Open-mindedness

It is probably true that most of us think we are fairly open-minded (unless we live within a particular religious or other type of culture that teaches adherence to a particularly strict code of conduct). If we stay open-minded we are slightly less likely to judge other people and automatically expect them to think and act as we do. To be open-minded, we must suspend the role of the 'adjudicator' that sits inside our heads telling us that something is good or something is bad – as referred to earlier.

One of the biggest problems in attempting to be open-minded is that we often do not know about the areas in which we are closed-minded. It is not until we are faced with situations we have not faced before that we realise that we are not quite as open-minded as we thought we were. We often do not know our own prejudices, especially when it comes to other people. Similarly, we are often open-minded in an 'arm's length' sort of way. There is an expression used in the UK – nimby – meaning 'not in my back yard'. When a new facility for, say, AIDS patients, those with mental health or drug issues is planned, even the most apparently open-minded sometimes suddenly find that they are not really as open-minded as they believed. It is OK for these sorts of facilities to be built 'somewhere', but I don't really want one 'in my back yard'.

Question for reflection

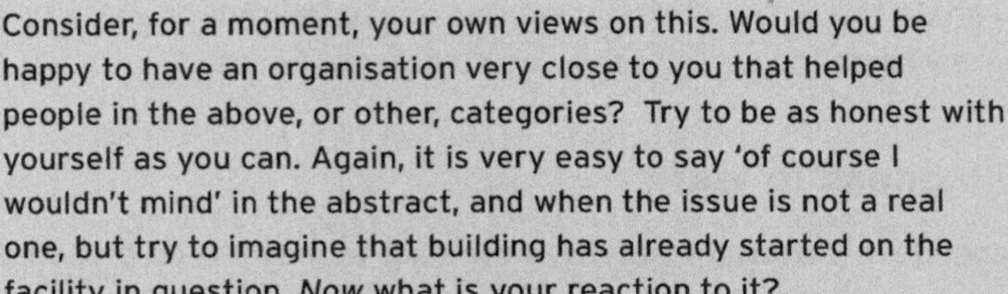

Consider, for a moment, your own views on this. Would you be happy to have an organisation very close to you that helped people in the above, or other, categories? Try to be as honest with yourself as you can. Again, it is very easy to say 'of course I wouldn't mind' in the abstract, and when the issue is not a real one, but try to imagine that building has already started on the facility in question. *Now* what is your reaction to it?

On a more personal level, we can learn much about people from other cultures if we show an open-minded curiosity towards them. By this I do not mean that we need to be nosy, but simply that we should meet them without preconceptions: we do not assume anything about them. Instead, we meet them afresh and find out who they are as they reveal themselves to us.

Interest in other people

It might be assumed that, almost by definition, nurses are interested in other people, but there seems to be no reason to assume that this is automatically true. Becoming culturally aware means that sometimes we have to try to forget ourselves and listen to the person we are encountering, with genuine interest (Andrews and Boyle, 2007). Yet listening is hard: it is difficult to really listen to another person for very long without some degree of judgement or disagreement. It is possible, however, to practise the art and skill of listening in a non-judgemental way, and this can be taught. Most student nurses are now taught interpersonal and listening skills as part of their educational programmes. It is important to continue to practise these skills throughout your career. There may even be a trajectory here: perhaps, as young people, we start by being self-interested and only interested in others as they relate to ourselves and our ways of thinking. As we get older, perhaps we lose some of this interest in self and give ourselves more completely to others, particularly if we have partners and children. Finally, as we get older, we may again become more self-interested as our social lives reduce.

For the purpose of developing cultural awareness, we *have* to be interested in others if we are to understand them (Helman, 2001), and not just in the sense of curiosity. We must want to know them as they are. If we can do this - really take an interest in people from other cultures - we are well on the way to achieving cultural awareness.

Willingness to learn

To engage in **culturally sensitive nursing**, we have to be prepared to learn about others (Papadopoulos, 2006, Andrews and Boyle, 2007). Most of us are trained in a particular style of nursing, i.e. that of the culture in which we live. As discussed, there are many other ways of nursing, just as there are many ways of communicating with others. It is important to be open to learning from others about their cultures and to be prepared to question and read. The theme of this book has been that 'ours is not the only culture', and once we begin to learn how other people do things, it can change our own lives and our own views of our culture. In learning about others, we learn about ourselves (Helman, 2001).

Lack of prejudice

Finally, in this short discussion about developing **cultural sensitivity**, we need to consider confronting our own prejudices. We all have them. We nearly all think that our way of doing things is 'right', and that other people, coming to the country in which we work, should learn as quickly as possible how things work in this country and adopt the styles and attitudes of people here. As we have seen, it is not as simple as that. Enculturation starts when we are very young (Lewis, 1985). We are taught how to do things, and how to act in relation to others. Simply coming to another country to work does not mean that we can somehow throw off all that learning and substitute for it the culture that we find ourselves in. Similarly, as residents, born and bred in the present culture, we should acknowledge that others coming to work here will think, communicate and do things differently.

One way to confront personal prejudices is to first of all acknowledge them, and then turn them on their heads. What would it be like if we thought the opposite of what we feel at the moment? Consider the following questions and reflect on your attitudes towards them. Try, if you can, to imagine yourself differently and in relation to each of the issues raised.

- If you are a Christian, what would it be like to be Muslim?
- If you are a Muslim, what would it be like to be Christian?
- If you are an unbeliever, what would it be like to believe in God?
- If you are straight, what would it be like to be gay?
- If you are gay, what would it be like to be straight?
- What if it was more normal to be gay than straight?
- If you were not a nurse, what would you be?
- If you are white, what would it be like to be brown or black?
- If you are brown or black, what would it be like to be white?
- If you say please and thank you a great deal, what would it be like *not* to say those things?
- If you do not say please and thank you very much, what would it be like to say them frequently?
- If you feel that men are superior to women in any way at all, what would it be like to feel the reverse?
- If you feel that women are superior to men in any way at all, what would it be like to feel the reverse?

Consider your most deeply held beliefs about you, your family, your religion (or lack of it), your community and your country, and try, for just a few minutes, to consider what it would be like not to hold those views. It is only by going beneath the surface of our everyday lives that we can uncover the prejudices we hold. Although we cannot expect to throw off our own cultural conditioning, we can at least try.

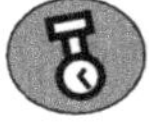

Challenging others

It is not uncommon to hear racial remarks, or remarks that belittle other people's cultures. Where we can, we should be prepared to confront them. One relatively easy way of dealing with this is not to respond to racist or anticultural jokes that others may tell us, or to point out that such jokes are inappropriate. This is not to suggest that we have to learn how not to have a sense of humour, but to appreciate that, to many, certain sorts of jokes and comments are simply not funny or, more worryingly, are hurtful or even dangerous: they may convey the idea that those from other cultures are 'in the wrong'. As we have seen, there are few if any absolute cultural rights and wrongs. Perhaps one of the few is that almost all cultures believe that we should treat others as we would like to be treated. This is known in philosophy as the **Golden Rule**. Clearly, if we make racist remarks or encourage them by responding to them when others make them, we are not adhering to this Golden Rule. If we are truly to become multicultural in our attitudes and actions, we must start by looking very closely at ourselves. We will never be entirely free of prejudice, and nor will other people. We can, however, do our best to overcome these negative attributes and encourage others to do the same. Bear in mind, too, that in many countries, including the UK, racist and anticultural remarks and ways of treating others are not only frowned upon but also illegal, and that others can take action against us if we are blatantly racist. This, however, is not the point. If we are interested in caring for the whole person and for caring for anyone, wherever they come from and whatever they believe, then we should *want* to discard our prejudices towards others, and should be actively involved in helping others to face theirs.

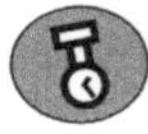

Transcultural nursing

Transcultural nursing is essentially an amalgam of anthropology and nursing, and, like many other nursing concepts, emerged from North America in around the late 1950s and early 1960s (Leininger, 1991). The movement, particularly in the United States, is based largely on the premise that nurses who work in multicultural societies are proficient in discovering and using pertinent cultural information so that they can better provide 'culturally sensitive and appropriate nursing care' (Mulhall, 1994).

In the UK, however, there has generally been far less research and debate regarding transcultural nursing. Only since the 1980s has there been a significant increase in the publications of articles on this subject in UK nursing journals (Mulhall, 1994, Papadopoulos, 2006). The discipline has recently grown in popularity in many countries, largely because of increasing multiculturalism. A critique of the movement is beyond the scope of this book, but readers who wish to know more about transcultural issues and transcultural nursing (particularly how it can inform nursing practice) are advised to explore some of the suggested reading material.

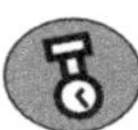

Closing thoughts

The purpose of this book is to (hopefully) raise awareness of the potential impact that culture and cultural issues can have on nursing and communication within nursing practice. Undoubtedly, many readers would prefer more specific, detailed information about the beliefs, practices and behaviours of particular cultural and/or religious groups that could be used to inform practice. However, as stated at the outset, such a 'tick box' approach was deliberately avoided, for several reasons.

First, it is simply impossible to know every individual cultural background (Andrews and Boyle, 2007). Second, such an approach would present a rather 'static' concept of particular cultures that did not account for variations between and within cultures. As discussed earlier, all cultures are in a constant process of evolution and change, owing to a variety of factors (migration, political and financial climates, social factors and so on). Finally, there is a danger that providing such specific information could result in the generalisation of certain cultures or religious groups, and possibly lead to stereotyping, labelling, misunderstandings, prejudices and even discrimination (Helman, 2001).

Any information or advice provided in this or any other book should ideally be used as a tentative starting point to facilitate the nurse's understanding of patients' cultural beliefs. However, they should never be relied upon to provide the 'absolute truth', and they should always be considered along with the patients' personal perspectives. Engaging with, and learning from, patients and colleagues from other cultures is therefore recommended, as and when appropriate.

Obviously there is much work to be done, particularly at an educational level, if nurses are to truly provide culturally sensitive health care (Andrews and Boyle, 2007). Improvements in pre- and post-registration nurse education and training in the UK in transcultural competence are required, along with further research in the area. For example, areas that need to be addressed include curriculum design, teaching and learning methods and content, and who should be responsible for teaching the nurses (e.g. nurses specially trained in transcultural issues, and/or an interdisciplinary approach involving anthropologists) (Andrews and Boyle, 2007). Further research is required at both clinical and educational levels, in order to establish how best to learn, teach and train nurses to care for patients from other cultures. There can be little doubt, however, that developing transcultural nursing in the UK requires a commitment to a set of clearly identified and agreed values, as well as appropriate teacher development, resources and organisation systems to support and promote such a philosophy (Papadopoulos, 2006). Undoubtedly, providing culturally appropriate nursing care is very challenging and will require a great deal of thought, caring concern and a willingness to learn from those we nurse (Dobson, 1991).

Suggested reading

Andrews MM and Boyle JS (2007). *Transcultural Concepts in Nursing Care,* 5th edn. Baltimore: Lippincott, Williams & Wilkins.

Helman C (2007). *Culture, Health and Illness,* 5th edn. London: Hodder Arnold.

Papadopoulos I (2006). *Transcultural Health and Social Care: Development of Culturally Competent Practitioners.* Oxford: Churchill Livingstone.

Glossary

Agnostic An agnostic is either someone who believes that any discussion of God is a waste of time, as no proof of his or her existence can ever be identified, or someone who is uncertain about the existence or otherwise of God.

Anthropology Anthropology is the academic study of humans, in a social context. Anthropologists study the ways in which people live together in groups. In the past, they used to focus mostly on 'exotic' societies (or those societies that are different from those in the west). Increasingly, anthropologists have come to study aspects of their own 'home-grown' cultures.

Assessment Assessment is the judgement, by a teacher, of a student's progress on an academic course. It may involve examinations, written work or oral investigations. The term should not be confused with *evaluation*.

Atheist An atheist is usually someone who, given any evidence to the contrary, believes that God does not exist. More radical forms of atheism may hold that believing in God is not only ludicrous but also potentially harmful.

Attending Attending is an extension of listening. It is 'being present' for the other person. It is offering complete concentration on the other person. When we are not 'attending' we are often only half listening to the other person, and engaging in an unrelated internal dialogue in our own heads.

Belief and truth Belief is holding something to be true. Truth is a fact about the world. No amount of believing something can make it true.

Collectivist societies A phrase sometimes used by anthropologists and sociologists to denote societies in which the family group is deemed more important than the individual. Examples of collectivist cultures include many in Asia, particularly South-east Asia. In collectivist societies there is great emphasis on respect for the family and for collective decision-making, and much less emphasis on the 'self'. The term is often associated with eastern cultures.

Communication Communication, as used in this book, involves both the verbal and non-verbal aspects of telling our story to others and hearing their responses. We cannot *not* communicate. We communicate through speech, the ways in which we use language and words, as well as through our facial expressions and other forms of non-verbal exchange.

Cultural awareness Cultural awareness is the ability to understand other cultures, acquired by reading, being taught or - most particularly - by visiting or living in other countries and cultures.

Cultural outsider A cultural outsider is someone visiting (or living in) a culture that is different from his or her own. The experience may be both helpful and not so helpful. On the one hand, the outsider may see cultural differences that are taken for granted by the insider. On the other hand, the outsider may simply not understand some cultural behaviours in the 'different' culture.

Cultural pitfalls Cultural pitfalls are those made through ignorance of cultural behaviour. For example, in many eastern cultures it is considered rude for a person to sit with their legs crossed. This poses a potential pitfall for the person who does not know of this rule.

Cultural sensitivity In this book, cultural sensitivity has been used to express the idea of our being aware of the various ways in which people live together in cultures. It can be encouraged by deep reading on the topic, through open-mindedness, through visiting other countries and cultures, and by listening to those from other cultures and accepting what they say.

Culturally sensitive nursing Culturally sensitive nursing is where people are cared for by a nurse who fully appreciates cultural differences and subtleties and who does not try to impose their prevailing culture onto the patient.

Culture Simply stated, culture refers to the ways in which a given society lives together. It includes references to beliefs, behaviours, routines, rituals, and the things that a society deems to be the appropriate way to live.

Culture shock Culture shock is the experience that a person has when becoming immersed, usually for the first time, in a culture in which many of the norms are completely different from those held in their own culture. For example, a North American who goes to live in Japan may experience culture shock through not fully understanding the differences between the USA and Japanese cultures.

Direct and indirect communication In western cultures, communication is often direct (e.g. 'Can you do this for me, please?' 'No, I am sorry, I cannot'). In eastern cultures communication may be more circular and less direct (e.g. 'Can you do this for me, please?' 'That may be a little difficult.') The use of indirect communication is often linked to *face* and the desire for people to ensure that neither party loses dignity or self-esteem.

Discrimination In this sense, to discriminate is to act negatively towards someone because of their sex, age, race, culture or any other variable. We discriminate against elderly patients, for example, if we believe that they are all somehow less intellectually bright than their younger counterparts.

Empathy Empathy is the ability to 'put yourself in someone else's shoes'. It is the ability to understand what another person is feeling, without relating what they are feeling back to your own experience.

Ethnocentrism The tendency to believe that the culture in which one is born and/or lives is the 'right' culture. To be ethnocentric is to believe that other people in the world should live as one does oneself. Ethnocentrism is perhaps a hugely difficult thing to avoid. Given that each of us is born into and grows up in a particular culture means that our own way of life is deeply ingrained within us. However, if we are really going to understand and respect other cultures, we have to find ways of rising above being ethnocentric.

Ethnography Ethnography is a qualitative research method in which the researcher studies the ways in which people live in a particular culture. The ethnographer may use personal observations, conversations, reflections, texts and other methods of gathering information about the culture.

Evaluation To evaluate something is to place a value on it. Evaluation involves inviting people to express their thoughts and feelings about how good or bad they perceived an experience or a course to be.

Existential moment This is the moment at which a child or adolescent may suddenly realise that he or she can think for themselves, and that they are not bound by what their parents or teachers tell them.

Eye contact Eye contact is a cultural variable. In many western societies it is expected that both parties in a conversation will maintain steady but comfortable eye contact. In many Asian and Islamic cultures, it is sometimes held that it is unacceptable for a 'junior' person to make regular eye contact with a 'senior' person. Similarly, eye contact between the sexes may vary considerably between cultures.

Face 'Face' is a concept often associated with Asian cultures. It involves the idea of being respected and showing respect to others. To 'lose face', or to suffer from 'broken face', is to experience a sudden or gradual loss of respect. Many Asian people will work hard to avoid both losing face and causing others to lose it.

Four Noble Truths The basis of the Buddhist religion. Although translations of the Four Noble Truths, from ancient documents, can vary, they are often described as follows:

1. All life is suffering.
2. Suffering is caused by attachment (to things and people).
3. There is a way of escaping from suffering.
4. The way of escaping from suffering is by following the Eightfold Path.

In turn, the Eightfold Path offers a prescription for living and involves the following:

1. Right view
2. Right intention
3. Right speech
4. Right action
5. Right livelihood
6. Right effort
7. Right mindfulness
8. Right concentration.

Gesture Gesture, in human communication, refers to both the amount and type of hand and arm movements made during conversation. There are huge cultural variations in its use, and the person who wants to become culturally sensitive needs to study such gestures carefully. In some Asian cultures very few hand gestures are used, as they are considered either rude or lacking in self-control. In many Latin cultures, gesture is used routinely as something that 'supports' the spoken word. It should be noted that in some cultures certain gestures are considered insulting, and that these gestures are not *universally* viewed in this way. It is important to know which gestures are acceptable and which are not, in any given culture.

Glass ceiling This phrase is used to indicate that women often fail to be promoted to a high level, or to earn salaries equal to those earned by men.

Golden Rule The Golden Rule is a moral rule from philosophy which can be summed up by the expression that we should treat others as we would wish to be treated. Variants of it exist in most major religious texts.

Individualist societies A phrase sometimes used by anthropologists and sociologists to denote societies in which the individual is deemed to be important. In individualist societies there is usually great emphasis on the 'self' and on achieving 'personal goals'. The term is often associated with western cultures.

In loco parentis This Latin phrase means roughly 'standing in for parents'. In the UK and USA, primary and secondary school teachers are substitute parents in the view of the law, but this is not the case in further education. In Thailand, however, a university teacher is also *in loco parentis* in relation to their students. These facts change the ways in which eastern and western university staff and lecturers interact with each other. In western universities, relationships are usually fairly casual. In eastern universities they are often very formal.

Lecture A lecture is usually a formal presentation of information, by a teacher, from the front of a classroom or lecture theatre.

Listening Listening, in human communication, involves more than simply 'hearing the words'. It also involves an ability to understand the meaning of what is being said. It is usually helpful for a person who is listening and who is not sure of the meaning, to clarify that meaning with the speaker.

Listening behaviours Listening behaviours are those that show the other person we are listening. Examples include facing the person, maintaining culturally sensitive eye contact, appropriate head nodding, and use of verbal markers that indicate that we are listening (e.g. 'yes . . .' '. . . certainly . . .' etc.).

Mai pen rai This is a Thai phrase roughly translated as 'It doesn't matter', or 'It's no problem'. It is used to smooth over slightly awkward social interactions and mistakes in order to help ensure that no one loses face.

Merit making Merit making is a Buddhist concept in which good actions are carried out to help ensure a higher level of rebirth in the next life, or simply because it is better to do good than not to do it.

Nationalism Nationalism is a deeply felt sense of pride for the country or culture into which a person is born. It is sometimes a variant of ethnocentricity and can lead people to believe that their own way of living is 'right', and that the ways in which others live are 'wrong'. At its most extreme it has led to major wars over the defence of one nation against another.

Phatic communication Phatic communication relates to all the aspects of spoken communication that are 'content free'. When we say 'Hello, how are you?', we are engaging in phatic communication: we are not enquiring about the other person's health, but merely indicating that we are friendly and open to conversation.

Proximity Proximity is the closeness or distance between two or more people when speaking. In Latin countries it is not unusual for people to stand very close to each other when speaking, and this may be accompanied by one speaker touching the other. In some Asian countries the comfortable distance between two speakers may be further apart, and no touching may take place.

Qualitative research Qualitative research sets out to explore people's views, beliefs and attitudes. Among other methods used to collect data it relies on interviews, observations, reflections and diary keeping.

Racism Racism is (usually an intense) dislike of others, based on race. It is another variation of ethnocentrism, in which a person believes that their own culture, nation or skin colour makes them superior to others. It has been the cause of extreme prejudice, personal attack and even wars. It has also led to those affected by it losing a number of their human rights.

Religion Religion is usually a formalised set of beliefs about the nature and existence of God (or gods) and an afterlife. Exceptions to this are religions such as Buddhism, which do not contain a concept of God.

Sanuk *Sanuk* is a Thai word that roughly means 'fun'. In Thai culture it is an important concept, and some have commented that in Thailand nothing is worth doing unless it is *sanuk*.

Seminar A seminar is usually a meeting of a small group of students with a lecturer or teacher, in which one or more of the students will make a presentation to the group. The presentation is then discussed by everyone in the group.

Six Category Intervention Analysis Six Category Intervention Analysis is a format devised by the British philosopher and humanistic psychologist John Heron to identify a range of useful and helpful communication skills. He suggests that, in order to help other people, we can choose to be *prescriptive*, *informative*, *confronting*, *cathartic*, *catalytic* or *supportive*. Heron claims that we can use these categories of communication to guide our intentions in any given helpful conversation. For more details, see Chapter 3.

Spirituality Spirituality is a rather vague word that incorporates not only formal beliefs about God and religion but also other, 'New Age' forms.

Stereotyping Stereotyping, in a cultural context, occurs when we treat people who look or act a certain way as necessarily being the same. For example, if a person from the UK believes that all Chinese people are 'similar', then that person is stereotyping. Similarly, if a person thinks that all gay people are much the same, that person is engaging in stereotypical thinking. Stereotyping does little to help us understand people.

Touch As indicated under ***Proximity***, the degree to which one speaker may touch another is governed by cultural norms. In Islamic societies, for example, it may be unacceptable for a man to touch a woman during a conversation. As noted above, in Latin countries, such as Spain or Italy, it may be quite routine for people to touch one another as they speak.

Traditional medicine Traditional medicine can be compared and contrasted with 'modern' medicine (by which is usually also meant western medicine). It is the medicine practised by healers and other gifted or especially knowledgeable local people, - particularly in rural areas.

Transcultural nursing Transcultural nursing is essentially an amalgam of anthropology and nursing, and like many other nursing concepts, emerged from North America in around the late 1950s and early 1960s (Leininger, 1991). The movement, particularly in the United States, is based largely on the premise that nurses who work in multicultural societies are proficient in discovering and using pertinent cultural information so that they can better provide 'culturally sensitive and appropriate nursing care' (Mulhall, 1994).

Turn-taking Turn-taking refers to the ways in which two or more people do or do not allow others to finish what they are saying. In some cultures, such as the USA and UK, the tendency is for people to 'take turns' in their utterances. However, in other cultures, for example Thai, it is not uncommon for people to speak at the same time. This is not an indicator of politeness or rudeness, merely a sign of cultural difference.

Tutorial A tutorial is normally a one-to-one educational meeting between a lecturer and a student.

Unbeliever An unbeliever is similar to an atheist and is someone who does not believe in God (or in gods).

Value sets In this book, the term 'value set' is used to indicate the ways in which different cultures list their values, and how those lists can vary according to where in the world a person lives.

References

Agar MH (2006). *The Professional Stranger*. San Diego: Academic Press.

Allen D (1998). Record keeping and routine nursing practice: the view from the wards. *Journal of Advanced Nursing* **27:** 1223-1230.

Andrews MM and Boyle JS (2007). *Transcultural Concepts in Nursing Care*, 5th edn. Baltimore: Lippincott, Williams & Wilkins.

Barbour RS (2001). Checklists for improving rigour in qualitative research: a case of the tail wagging the dog? *British Medical Journal* **322:** 1115-1117.

Barnard A and Spencer J (2002). *Encyclopaedia of Social and Cultural Anthropology*. London: Routledge.

Bowker J (2006). *World Religions*. London: Dorling Kindersley.

Brown P and Levinson S (1987). *Politeness: some Universals in Language*. Cambridge: Cambridge University Press.

Bruni N (1988). A critical analysis of transcultural theory. *Australian Journal of Advanced Nursing* **5 (3):** 26-32.

Burden B (1998). Privacy or help? The use of curtain positioning strategies within the maternity ward environment as a means of achieving and maintaining privacy, or as a form of signalling to peers and professionals in an attempt to seek information or support. *Journal of Advanced Nursing* **27:** 15-23.

Burnard P (1991). A method of analysis of interview transcripts in qualitative research. *Nurse Education Today* **11:** 461-466.

Burnard P (1998). Personal qualities or skills? A report of a study of nursing students' views of the characteristics of counsellors. *Nurse Education Today* **18:** 649-654.

Burnard P (2002). *Learning Human Skills: an Experiential Guide for Nurses and Health Care Professionals*, 4th edn. Oxford: Butterworth-Heineman.

Burnard P (2004). Writing a qualitative research report. *Nurse Education Today* **24:** 174-179.

Burnard P and Gill P (2007). The heresy of the 'recent' reference [editorial]. *Nurse Education Today* **27 (7):** 665-666.

Burnard P and Morrison P (1988). Nurses' perceptions of their interpersonal skills: a descriptive study using Six Category Intervention Analysis. *Nurse Education Today* **8:** 266–272.

Burnard P and Naiyapatana W (2004). *Culture and Communication in Thai Nursing.* Cardiff: University of Wales College of Medicine.

Burnard P Edwards D Bennet K *et al.* (2008). A comparative, longitudinal study of stress in student nurses in five countries: Albania, Brunei, the Czech Republic, Malta and Wales. *Nurse Education Today* **28:** 134–145.

Carson J and Kuipers E (1998). Stress management interventions. In: Hardy S, Carson J and Thomas B, eds. *Occupational Stress: Personal and Professional Approaches.* Cheltenham: Stanley Thornes.

Collins J (2002). *High-pop: Making Culture into Popular Entertainment.* Chichester: WileyBlackwell.

Coser LA (1977). *Masters of Sociological Thought: Ideas in Historical and Social Context*, 2nd edn. NewYork: Harcourt Brace.

Cutcliffe JR and McKenna HP (1999). Establishing the credibility of qualitative research findings: the plot thickens. *Journal of Advanced Nursing* **30:** 374–380.

Davis H and Fallowfield L (eds) (1991). *Counselling and Communication in Health Care*. Chichester: Wiley.

Dawkins R (2006). *The God Delusion*. London: Black Swan.

Dobson SM (1991). *Transcultural Nursing.* London: Scutari.

Dodd CH (1991). *Dynamics of Intercultural Communication*, 3rd edn. Dubuque: Brown.

Egan G (1982). *The Skilled Helper,* 2nd edn. Monterey, CA: Brooks/Cole.

Ekachai S (2002). *Keeping the Faith: Thai Buddhism at the Crossroads.* Bangkok: Post Books.

Ellsworth PC (1994). Sense, culture and sensibility. In: Kitayama S and Markus RH, eds. *Emotion and Culture: Empirical Studies of Mutual Influence*. Washington, DC: American Psychological Association.

Evans-Pritchard EE (1962). *Social Anthropology* and other essays. New York: The Free Press.

Evans-Pritchard EE (1966). *Theories of Primitive Religion*. Oxford: Clarendon Press.

Fox K (2005). *Watching the English*. London: Hodder and Stoughton.

Frederickson J (2003). The eclipse of the person in psychoanalysis. In: Frie R ed. *Understanding Experience: Psychotherapy and Postmodernism*. London: Routledge.

Frie R (ed.) (2003). *Understanding Experience: Psychotherapy and Postmodernism*. London: Routledge.

Ganeri A (1999). *My Hindu Faith*. London: Evans.

Gans HJ (1999). *Popular Culture and High Culture: An Analysis and Evaluation of Taste*. Jackson, FL: Basic Books Inc.

Gerrish K (1997). Preparation of nurses to meet the needs of an ethnically diverse society: educational implications. *Nurse Education Today* **17:** 359-365.

Gerrish K and Papadopoulos I (1999). Transcultural competence: the challenge for nurse education. *British Journal of Nursing* **8 (21):** 1453-1457.

Gill P (2000). Brainstem death - an anthropological perspective. *Care of the Critically Ill* **16 (6):** 217-220.

Gill P (2004). Difficulties in developing a nursing research culture in the UK. *British Journal of Nursing* **13 (14):** 876-879.

Gill P (2006). *Illuminating donor and recipient experiences in live kidney transplantation*. Unpublished PhD Thesis, Cardiff University, Cardiff.

Gyatso GK (2001). *Introduction to Buddhism: An Explanation of the Buddhist Way of Life*. Cumbria: Tharpa Publications.

Hammersley M and Atkinson P (2007). *Ethnography: Principles in Practice*, 3rd edn. London: Routledge.

Hanvey RG (1979). Cross-cultural awareness. In: Smith EC and Fiber L Luce, eds. *Towards Internationalism*. Rowley, MA: Newbury House.

Hargie O, Saunders C and Dickson D (1994). *Social Skills in Interpersonal Communication*, 3rd edn. London: Routledge.

Harris M (1999). *Theories of Culture in Postmodern Times*. Walnut Creek, CA: AltaMira Press.

Harris S (2006). *The End of Faith: Religion, Terror, and the Future of Reason*. Glencoe: Free Press.

Harvey P (1990). *An Introduction to Buddhism: Teachings, History and Practices*. Cambridge: Cambridge University Press.

Hellweg SA, Samovar LA and Skow L (1991). Cultural variations in negotiation styles. In: Samovar LA and Porter M, eds. *Intercultural Communications: a reader*. Belmont: Wadsworth.

Helman CG (2001). *Culture, Health and Illness,* 4th edn. Oxford: Butterworth-Heinemann.

Hendry J (2008). *An Introduction to Social Anthropology: Sharing Our Worlds*, 2nd edn. Basingstoke: Palgrave Macmillan.

Heron J (1989). Six Category Intervention Analysis, 3rd edn. Human Potential Resource Group, University of Surrey, Guildford.

Hitchens C (2006). *God Is Not Great: The Case Against Religion*. London: Atlantic Books.

Hoffman E (1989). *Lost in Translation*. New York: Dutton.

Hofstede G (1994). *Culture and Organisations: Software of the Mind*. London: McGraw Hill.

Holland K (1999). A journey to becoming: the student nurse in transition. *Journal of Advanced Nursing* **29 (1):** 229–236.

Holloway I and Wheeler S (1996). *Qualitative Research for Nurses*. Oxford: Blackwell.

Hutchinson Encyclopaedia (2000). Oxford: Helicon Publishing.

Juethong W (1998). *Thai Baccalaureate Nursing Students' Caring and Uncaring: Lived Experience with Thai Nursing Instructors*. Unpublished PhD thesis. Fairfax, VA: George Mason University.

Klausner WJ (1993). *Reflections on Thai Culture: Collected Writings*. Bangkok: The Siam Society.

Kluckhohn C (1969). *Mirror For Man: The Relation of Anthropology to Modern Life*. New York: McGraw Hill.

Korzenny F (1991). Relevance and application of intercultural communication theory and research. In: Samovar LA and Porter M, eds. *Intercultural Communications: a reader*. Belmont, CA: Wadsworth.

Kuper A (1996). *Anthropology and Anthropologists: The Modern British School,* 3rd edn. London: Routledge.

Kvale S (1996). *Interviews: An Introduction to Qualitative Research Interviewing.* Thousand Oaks, CA: Sage Publications.

Leach E (1982). *Social Anthropology*. Oxford: Oxford University Press.

Leininger MM (1991). *Culture, Care, Diversity and Universality: A Theory of Nursing*. New York: National League of Nursing.

Lent JA (1995). *Asian Popular Culture*. Boulder, CO: Westview.

Lewis IM (1985). *Social Anthropology in Perspective,* 2nd edn. Cambridge: Cambridge University Press.

Linton R (1945). Present world conditions in cultural perspective. In: Linton R, ed. *The Science of Man in World Crisis.* New York: Columbia University Press, pp. 201-21.

Macqueen S (1995). Anthropology and germ theory. *Journal of Hospital Infection* **30 (Suppl.):** 116-126.

Madrid A (1994). Diversity and its discontents. In: Samovar LA and Porter RE, eds. *Intercultural Communication: a reader*. Belmont, CA: Wadsworth.

Malinowski B (1922). *Argonauts of the Western Pacific: an Account of Native Enterprise and Adventure in the Archipelago of Melanesian New Guinea.* London: Routledge.

Malinowski B (1923). The problem of meaning in primitive languages. In: Ogden CK and Richards IA, eds. *The Meaning of Meaning: A Study of the Influence of Language upon Thought and the Science of Symbolism.* London: Routledge & Kegan Paul.

Mays N and Pope C (1995). Rigour in qualitative research. *British Medical Journal* **311:** 109-19.

McLaren MC (1998). *Interpreting Cultural Differences: the Challenge of Intercultural Communication*. Dereham: Peter Francis.

McSherry W, Cash K and Ross L (2004). Meaning of spirituality: implications for nursing practice. *Journal of Clinical Nursing* **13:** 934-941.

Mills L-K. *Understanding Buddhism*. Chiang Mai: Silkworm.

Morrison P and Burnard P (1991). *Caring and Communicating: the Interpersonal Relationship in Nursing*, 2nd edn. Basingstoke: Macmillan.

Mulder N (2000). *Inside Thai Society: Religion, Everyday Life, Change.* ChiangMai: Silkworm.

Mulhall A (1994). Anthropology: a model for nursing. *Nursing Standard* **8 (31):** 35-38.

Nemetz Robinson G (1985). *Crosscultural Understanding: Processes and Approaches for Foreign Language, English as a Second Language and Bilingual Educators*. London: Pergamon.

Nichter M (1993). Social-science lessons from diarrhoea research and their application to ARI. *Human Organization* **52 (1):** 53-67.

Papadopoulos I (2006). *Transcultural Health and Social Care: Development of Culturally Competent Practitioners*. Oxford: Churchill Livingstone.

Papadopoulos I, Tilki M and Alleyne J (1994). Transcultural nursing and nurse education. *British Journal of Nursing* **3 (11):** 583-586.

Parahoo K (2006). *Nursing Research: Principles, Processes and Issues*, 2nd edn. Basingstoke: Palgrave Macmillan.

Rapport N and Overing J (2006). *Social and Cultural Anthropology: The Key Concepts*. London: Routledge.

Said E (1979). *Orientalism*. New York: Random House.

Sapir E (1948). Culture, language, genuine and spurious. In: Maudelbaum DG, ed. (1960) Edward Sapir: *Culture, Language and Personality*. Selected essays. California: University of California Press, pp. 78–119.

Seaman A and Brown A (1999). *My Christian Faith*. London: Evans.

Silverman D (2000). *Doing Qualitative Research*. London: Sage.

Smart N (1998). *The World's Religions*, 2nd edn. Cambridge: Cambridge University Press.

Sumner WG (1906). *Folkways*. Boston, MA: Ginn.

Swendson C and Windsor C (1996). Rethinking cultural sensitivity. *Nursing Inquiry* **3:** 3–10.

Tomlinson J (2000). Cultural imperialism. In: Lechuer FJ and Boli J, eds. *The Globalization Reader*. Oxford: Blackwell, pp. 307–315.

Triandis HC (1972). Collectivism v. individualism. In: Gudykunst WB and Kim YY, eds. *Readings on Communicating with Strangers*. New York: McGraw Hill.

Triandis HC, Brislin R and Hui CH (1991). Cross-cultural training across the individualism–collectivism divide. In: Samovar P and Porter D, eds. *Individual Communication: a reader*, 6th edn. Belmont, CA: Wadsworth.

Valdes JM (1986). *Culture Bound: Readings for Writers*. New York: St Martin's Press.

Van der Geest S (1995). Overcoming ethnocentrism: How social science and medicine relate and should relate to one another. *Social Science and Medicine* **40:** 869–872.

Varner I and Beamer L (1995). *Intercultural Communication in the Global Workplace*. Chicago: Irwin.

Wanguri DM (1996). Diversity, equity and communicative openness. *Journal of Business Communication* **33 (4):** 443–54.

Watzlawick P (1984). *The Invented Reality: how to we know what we know? Contributions to constructivism*. New York: Norton.

Weiss MG (1988). Conceptual models of diarrhoeal illness: conceptual framework and review. *Social Science and Medicine* **27 (1):** 5–16.

Weiss MG (1988). Conceptual models of diarrhoeal illness: conceptual framework and review. *Social Science and Medicine* **27 (1):** 5-16.

Wengraf T (2001). *Qualitative Research Interviewing: Biographic Narrative and Semi-structured Networks*. London: Sage.

Weston D *et al.* (2005). *Islam in Today's World*. London: Hodder Murray.

Wittgenstein L, trans. Pears DF and McGuinness BF (1966). *Tractatus Logico-Philosophicus.* London: Routledge Kegan Paul.

Index

N.B. Items listed in the Glossary are indicated by **bold** page numbers, case studies by [CS], and introductory text by roman numerals.

A

B

C

D

E

F

G

H

N

O

P

Q

R

S

T

U

V

W